PEBBLE IN THE BROOK:
RehabDramatics and the Engagement of Drama Therapy in Nigeria

PEBBLE IN THE BROOK:
RehabDramatics and the Engagement of Drama Therapy in Nigeria

Chukwudi Michael Okoye

GALDA VERLAG 2023

Bibliografische Information der Deutschen Nationalbibliothek
Die Deutsche Nationalbibliothek verzeichnet diese Publikation in der Deutschen Nationalbibliografie; detaillierte bibliografische Daten sind im Internet über https://dnb.de abrufbar.

Originally presented as the author's dissertation (doctoral) :
Nnamdi Azikiwe University, Awka, 2020

ISBN 978-3-96203-316-3 (Print)
ISBN 978-3-96203-317-0 (E-Book)

TABLE OF CONTENT

DEDICATION

For Nasiah, an inspiration, an Amazon, the wife of my youth.

And

The Management and pupils of the School for the Visually Impaired (formerly school for the Blind) Ivbiore, Edo State., The management and children of the Salvation Army, East Circular, Benin, Edo state. The management and students of God's Care Special School, Amaenyi, Awka, Anambra State and Management and patients of the Psychiatric Hospital Nawfia, Anambra State.

Let their stories be told. Let them be heard.

ACKNOWLEDGEMENTS

I am a product of God's grace and mercy. His Holy spirit has been my guide in more ways that I can recount; this book inclusive. To Him be all the Glory.

To my beloved parents, Reverend Apostle Peter & Evang. Mrs Ifeoma Okoye, I lack words to appreciate you for the support system you provided me with these years. I love you both.

I am deeply grateful to my teacher, Prof Tracie Utoh-Ezeajugh for her immense contributions, guidance and motherly disposition towards me especially while supervising my PhD which has given rise to the birth of this book; Words alone cannot describe how grateful I am to you for always finding time, despite your incredibly busy schedule, in providing rare Academic mentorship. I will always cherish you. I am also very grateful for the qualitative contributions of late Professor Canice Nwosu, late Professor Tina Okoye, Professor Alex Asigbo, Professor Charles Emeka Nwadigwe, Professor Agatha Onwuekwe, and Professor Isaac Nwankwo; all the constructive corrections I got from these brilliant minds provided me with needed "ammunition" to improve my research capability significantly and ultimately write this book. I am also grateful for the mentorship provided by late Professor Chiduo Obadiegwu who was a towering figure in the study of Theatre for Development in Nigeria and who also laid the foundation for research possibilities in the study of Applied theatre in the department of Theatre and Film studies, Nnamdi Azikiwe University, Awka.

I am also deeply grateful to the management and pupils of School for the Visually Impaired (formerly school for the Blind) Ivbiore, Edo State., The management and children of the Salvation Army center for Children with Disabilities, East Circular, Benin, Edo state. The management and students of God's Care Special School, Amaenyi, Awka, Anambra State and the Management and inmates of the Psychiatric Hospital, Nawfia, Anambra State, for giving me rare access to their facilities in the course of this research. It is my hope that this study will indeed open new vistas of learning that would give needed attention to the plight of challenged children and young adults in Nigeria.

To my spiritual mentors, Psts Obi and Azo Ogbo, Senior Pastors of Garden of Grace Church International, Awka, under whom I serve; Thank you so much for believing in me and showing me deep truths. I honour you.

To my friend and brother, Dr. Chima Agazue of the University of Huddersfield, United Kingdom, who literarily opened up his library and granted me unfettered access to helpful materials. God bless you.

I am also thankful for the assistance offered me by many individuals in the course of the work; Mr. Onome Otueroro, Mrs. Blessing Idede, Hon. Mrs. Gbinigie Florence, Engr. and Mrs. Kodichi. C., Ezeanyim, Hon. Princess Bibiana Ijeoma Nwankwo, Major Bramwell Chukwunwem, Dr. C. C. Onuorah, Mr. Kunle Adewale and others too numerous to mention. To my 400 level 2018/2019 "specialization" students namely; Osang Ruth Bunmi, Akachukwu Samuel Eze, Praise Etune Okafoanyali, Loveth Obum Ugwu, Sharon Nora Aneboh, Margaret Chetachi Luke, Chukwubusonma Ezelum, Hilda Amara Ezeude, Silvia Tochukwu Abazu, Martins Arinze Nwafor and Kingsley Chike Ekemezie, who were my research assistants in the *Nawfia* and *Amaenyi* Projects, I am most grateful.

Finally, of particular mention is my incredible wife, His worship, (Mrs.) Ifeyinwa Nasiah Okoye and my Children, Chukwukaima, Chukwudumaga and Chukwuzuelum who have had to bear the brunt of many "disappearing acts", "book dumps" and "mood swings" these past years during the course of putting this work together. I love you guys dearly. Your prayers and sacrifices have made this come to pass!

Chukwudi Michael Okoye

AUTHOR'S NOTE

At the onset of my Ph.D research in 2015, I was faced with the dilemma of where to pitch my research tent. Indeed, I am one of those who strongly believe that every research should be geared towards improving humanity, even if the outcome of the research would have a 0.01% impact: in my view, a positive endeavour, no matter how small, is a credible endeavour none the less.

Thus, this is the inspiration behind the concept of RehabDramatics. Spurred on the numerous milestones achieved by my forebears in the area of Applied Theatre which basically speaks of the application and engagement of live theatrical performances in addressing societal needs as they arise per time, the role of the theatre continues to persist as an art form that mirrors humanity across periods.

Drama therapy, therefore, though not an entirely new area in the study of Applied Theatre, provides a particular opening to the engagement of Dramatic techniques in fostering rehabilitative possibilities as well as improving qualitative psychosocial awareness and interactions in participants.

In Nigeria today, the present circumstances as they surround children and young adults who are either physically challenged or are exposed to psychological challenges as a result of the menace posed by Drug Abuse as well as other vices, are real and far reaching.

On one side of this problem is the question of the proper educative interventions that would provide particular and child centered remedies to the learning needs of these disadvantaged individuals.

On the other side, is the question of the role and approach of host communities and government institutions in engaging cultural and religious norms for the benefit of these challenged individuals rather than for their disadvantage.

It is therefore hoped that like a *pebble in the brook*, this book would aid in unraveling and rediscovering the potential of drama in contributing and adding beauty to other aspects of the human endeavour such as public health, special needs education and community mobilization.

Happy reading

We must keep asking questions

....till we ask through

CM Okoye

4th December, 2021

INTRODUCTION

The concept of Child development will continue to evoke conversations and debates due to its dynamic nature. Scholars have overtime worked on different ideas and formats; on not only what should be learnt, as well as what is expected of the Teacher-facilitator in given situations, but also on the question of what environment is befitting for child learning and hollistic development. Indeed, these concepts may vary from race to race and from one cultural enclave to the other, but as is the case most times, are likely to have similar underlining features or even results. Theatre scholars and practitioners have continued to make contributions on the use of the Theatre in community engagements and human development. The question therefore, on whether theatrical activities can be used to address social ills, reform mundane norms and even educate young minds have been answered with postulations from Theatre scholars the world over; Fields of study such as Theatre in Education, Creative Dramatics and Classroom Drama are still being explored to shape the ideology of child development and learning using theatrical forms. Tony Jackson for instance speaks of the Theatre in Education programme as: "not a performance in schools, or a self-contained play, a one off event that is here today and gone tomorrow, but a coordinated and carefully structured pattern of activities, usually devised and researched by the company around a topic of relevance both to the school curriculum and to the children's own lives".

The Theatre also addresses psychological development in children from the educational perspective. Theatrical situations can be used to solve simple and complex problems as they relate to the immediate needs of the child. Nellie MaCaslin further corroborates this, stating that "Few adults would deny the importance of arts in the education of their Children. To enjoy the arts and appreciate the richness they can add to human life, some preparation is needed. For most children, the preparation is or should be given in school. In summary the theatre arts are the least difficult of the arts to implement, with the greatest potential for learning".

Indeed, there are other schools of thought that propose that the engagement of drama in education, while promoting a range of activities, allows for a learning experience both for the child and the teacher-facilitator to be unraveled. Thus, educators like Gavin Bolton believe that projects like Classroom drama has to do with the creation of an art form in a way that is significant for the participants in the art-making experience, such that something new is understood or something is newly understood. In other different studies where drama has been adjudged as a valuable tool for child education and psychosocial development such as; Development drama, Creative drama, Drama therapy, and Health humanities, the underlying factor remains that child learning and development is more effective where the process is participatory, that is, where the child is involved in the art making process. Indeed, as Nellie McCaslin puts it, "Through creative drama, an individual has a chance to develop and grow. This is also true of the group in which ideas are explored, evaluated, changed and used. As a group of any age works together under sensitive and skilled leadership, the members learn to accept, appreciate and stimulate each other".

Theatre informs that through art forms such as dance and drama, the young mind develops academically, morally and socially. The use of creative drama thus, exposes children not only in learning drama; but to learn through drama. Accordingly Charles Combs asserts that "While drama is informed by many of the ideas and practices of Theatre arts, it is principally valued as a learning medium rather than an art form and is governed and validated through criteria rather than aesthetics, informal drama's goals are based on pedagogical, developmental and learning theory as much or more than they are art based; its objectives are manifold, but they are all directed towards the growth and development of the participant rather than the entertainment or simulation of the observer".

From the above assertion, it appears that the use of creative drama provides an enabling environment for child learning and development and could be utilized as a viable instrument in bringing other art forms such as role playing, singing, dancing, improvisation, together in the learning process and to the consciousness of the developing child. As a relatively fully unengaged educational tool, this method of learning engages the child in a wholesome, creative and practical experience that deviates from the age long teacher/ pupil norm, where the child is said to be seen and not heard. The aim of Drama in Education thus, allows for the development of the child, socially, intellectually and psychologically as he grapples with the demands of formal Education or as Hoetker James puts it, "Drama increases creativity, originality, sensitivity, fluency, flexibility, emotional stability, cooperation and examination of moral attitudes, while developing communication skills and the appreciation of literature".

Thus, the concept of RehabDramatics also attempts to bridge the gap between the prospects for both rehabilitation and education to occur simultaneously. The term RehabDramatics is made up of two word components; *Rehab* and *Dramatics*. The word *Rehab* is derived from the noun, Rehabilitation or the verb rehabilitate. The Online Etymology Dictionary (2019) defines rehabilitation as "bringing back to a former condition after decay or damage and in part from the Medieval Latin word, *rehabilitatus* meaning to restore one's reputation or character in the eyes of others". Given these definitions it would appear that the term Rehabilitation could derive more in-depth meaning within contextual applications and constructs. The Online Etymology dictionary gives further clarifications in defining the application of the term within certain scenarios inclusive of, "To restore to good condition, operation, ability to work or the like; To restore to good condition, operation or management as a bankrupt business; To reestablish the good reputation of a person, one's character or name "and"; To restore to former capacity, standing, rank, rights or privileges".

Indeed, as a word being used across and beyond disciplines of medical nature and also capable of being jointly referenced with synonyms such as, to salvage, restore, recondition, reconstruct and refurbish, the word Rehabilitation provides as an adequate base term in evaluating discourses on individuals who are faced with some form of physical or learning disability or the other. Indeed, taking a hint from the Latin derivation, the contextual appreciation of the word, Rehabilitation extends beyond its application to the possibility of achieving total wholesomeness and restoration of full physical functions due to immediate disabilities and challenges caused by accidental mishaps, blunt force traumas and so on, but also envisages more abstract situations as in the cases of secondary disabilities such as psychosocial challenges which primary physical disabilities may engender. The British Dictionary concurs with this position with the contextual definition of the verb, Rehabilitate as the ability "to help a person who has acquired a disability or addiction or who has just been released from prison. To readapt to society or a new job, as by vocational guidance, restraining or therapy".

Thus, as the studies carried out and documented within this book would show, there appears a need, not only to restore and readapt individuals who suffer from different disabilities back to society, but also to improve prospects for psychosocial development to thrive.

On the other word component, the Merriam-Webster Dictionary (2019) defines *Dramatics* as "the study and practice of theatrical arts such as acting and stagecraft" (n.pag). It then connotes that the use of the word *dramatics*, informs of the performance and production of plays as well as other theatrical or staged events. Derived from the word 'Drama' which portends a portrayal of life, involving conflicts and emotions through action, dialogue and designed for performance, the word dramatics ensures that certain components needed to create a theatrical event must come together to allow for a proper appreciation and evaluation of the production's objective. Perhaps, it is in this light that the term could be used and engaged within other approaches that project the efficacy of performative elements and performances, in the understanding of working concepts. The concept of Creative Dramatics for example, provides for the engagement of the imaginative ability of children through the instrumentality of drama in working through set tasks that formal environments such as schools provide. Indeed in Andrew Johnson's words "Creative dramatics uses students' imagination and willingness to act or pretend as a means of reinforcing academic, emotional and interpersonal objectives".

Thus, the concept of RehabDramatics attempts the coming together and utilization of the dramatic, theatrical and performance based arts, beyond the purpose of task-solving but in stimulating psychosocial improvements within each participating individual such that could foster rehabilitative possibilities in areas of self imagery, self representation, self worth and social relationships. The infusion of these performances should therefore provide artistic content that can be identifiable and relatable to circumstances within which the participant live. The need to engage oral literature and performances within the creative process can be used to aid knowledge acquisition and rehabilitative tendencies as the medium must not appear to be delineated from the present realities of participating individuals. RehabDramatics could be engaged as an approach in the use of Drama as a medium capable of fostering Therapeutic and transformative changes. The broader concept of Drama Therapy have overtime engaged particular approaches in evaluating the various complexities of human and social behaviour as well as the need to develop avenues where artistic and performative processes can be used to improve cognitive and creative possibilities needed for qualitative psychosocial behaviour. Reknowned psychologist, Elmien Butler citing Enumah, Verhofstadt-Deneve, Boal and others, state that "Drama therapy can be defined as the systematic and intentional use of drama/ theatre to achieve psychological change and growth. Manifestations of drama in the field of therapy include psychodrama, social theatre, playback theatre and movement as a linguistic activity. Drama therapy acknowledges the relevance and interdependence of health and creativity in an approach to space and healing that is interdisciplinary".

RehabDramatics, thus could be engaged within these processes with particular reference to the engagement of indigenous, artistic and performative content that is capable of not only enhancing dramatic activity and engagement, but also increasing acceptability of same through relatable communication avenues that are essential in improving therapeutic possibilities. The engagement of oral indigenous art forms is critical to this concept as it portends that the immediate society of every individual, and by extension its norms, cultural practices, languages and traditions is capable of influencing individual perceptions and behavior of its citizens and thus, could be infused along with other dramatic activities and processes to engender new approaches that could foster positive rehabilitative change.

As an operational term and used within the boundaries of the applied theatre projects carried out and documented in this book, RehabDramatics could be defined as the engagement and utilization of the dramatic art medium beyond the spheres of learning and *conscientization*, in inducing rehabilitative possibilities through a controlled and pragmatic inclusion of activities that are creative, expressive, participatory and development-driven to the study of challenged individuals. RehabDramatics advocates for the use and integration of oral and performative art forms, literature, techniques and instruments prevalent within the community of research in the process of engendering performance based learning and thus fostering improved cognitive and psychosocial development as it concerns transformative engagements with challenged persons. The concept of RehabDramatics integrates these inclusive and performative components of Drama along with existing oral traditions and literature such as poetry, folklore, puppetry, dramatic representations, dance and games in an attempt to bridge the gap for the prospects of both learning and rehabilitation to occur simultaneously.

In order to fully deploy the concept of RehabDramatics, there is need to engage research approaches such as the Interpretative Phenomenological Analysis, IPA in underscoring how certain experiences could affect the psychosocial outlook of individuals and how the performing arts could be utilized as an interventionist medium. The Interpretative Phenomenological Analysis (IPA) is a research approach that offers insight into the experiences of individuals and how these experiences inform their perceptions on a given phenomenon. Originally domiciled in the study of psychology and introduced by Jonathan Smith, IPA is quite distinct from other approaches and is uniquely suitable in the discourse of Rehabilitative-Drama because of its Psychological, interpretative and idiographic components. Studies have overtime evaluated the potentiality of IPA in drama related concepts. Gabriela Dima, in the study for the inclusion of the method of interpretative phenomenological Analysis in Psychodrama research, submits that "studies Using IPA bring an in depth understanding and sense-making of the experiences of participants in various psychodrama groups, they reveal therapeutic change process and the personal meaning of therapeutic outcomes".

Indeed as a model of Drama therapy, RehabDramatics engages the participants in an art making process; where experiences are shared but made collaborative by the introduction of Dramatic enactments and oral traditional art forms such as Folklore, songs, games, etc. Susan Cassidy, while quoting the North American Drama Therapy Association, supports this position when she says that "Drama therapy is an active, experimental approach to facilitating change. Through story-telling, projective play, purposeful improvisation and performance, participants are invited to rehearse desired behaviors, practice being in relationships, expand and find flexibility between life roles, and perform the change they wish to be and see in the world".

The primary concept of the Interpretative Phenomenological Analysis in the context of this research, allows for a study that is flexible such that various artistic techniques and procedures could be adopted to suit each given situation. Dima, again acknowledging Smith's recommendation for the integration of IPA in psycho-dramatic exercises posits that "there is no single definitive way of doing IPA, but it offers clear guidance and suggestions for the analysis, interpretation and writing process; and also advice for researchers on how to adapt the method to their own particular way of working".

There is need, however, for proper guidelines to be drawn in the application of IPA. This ensures that a given progress pattern is observed and experiences are adequately taken note of and documented. Dima, suggests that "Consistent with IPA theoretical foundations, research tends to focus on people's experiences and/or understandings of a particular phenomena, on personal meaning and sense making in a particular context for people who share specific experiences, hence IPA is suitable to respond to broadly and openly framed research questions". Adequate authorizations and permissions should be sought to ensure credibility of the findings of the researcher. The research approach of IPA also thrives in an environment that is both conducive and safe for participants.

Indeed, the rehabilitative potential, of drama may not be as widely used as an approach within the Nigerian educational system even though it is also generally accepted that a percentage of Nigerian children do not undergo any form of formal education. Worse still is the indication that many children could be best described as "at risk", due to the debilitating environment they are being brought up in. It is not common for a Nigerian child even today to be diagnosed with ADHD (Attention Deficit Hyperactive Disorder), GAD (General Anxiety Disorder) or PTSD (Post Traumatic Stress Disorder), whereas the conditions that escalate these tendencies as well as other psychological deficiencies appear quite prevalent in Nigeria as they are around the world.

There are indications that the number of broken homes in Nigeria are on the increase. Worrisome still is the fact that many spouses now jettison the option of legally divorcing their partners by either just staying separated or even going ahead to marry someone else; thereby leaving the child or children born in the original union in very precarious situations. Robert Clarke, quoting the National Bureau of Statistics reports that "Official statistics suggest that divorce is exceedingly uncommon in Nigeria. Just 0.2% of men and 0.3% of women have legally untied the knot, according to the National Bureau of statistics. And well under 1% of couples admit to being separated yet such counts exclude the vast majority of Nigerians whose traditional marriage ceremonies are not governed by modern law".

In the instance where these marital issues are brought before the courts, it becomes even more evident that certain situations within the home could indeed trigger negative behavioral and psychological traits in children. The Immigration and Refugee Board of Canada, in a publication on Nigeria's Divorce law and practices, quotes Bambo Adesanya, SAN, in an attempt to underscore the Nigerian Judicial System's Contribution to the growing causes of divorce in Nigeria. It reports that "The types of behavior referred to include rape, sodomy, bestiality, habitual drunkenness or intoxication, misuse of drugs, frequent convictions, habitually leaving spouse without support, attempted murder, assaults, insanity, humiliating treatment, nagging and the use of juju (a charm or fetish). Adesanya adds that in a 1972 court ruling, habitual intemperate consumption of alcohol and inordinate sexual indulgences of the respondent with all sorts of women particularly housemaids were held to be weighty unreasonable acts to expect the petitioner to put up with".

Indeed, some other unhealthy circumstances at risk children are faced with, maybe through no fault or even active involvement of theirs or their parents. Children who are physically challenged, obese or suffer from biological or genetic disorders such as Down syndrome, Deafness, Albinism, Sickle cell Anemia, and Blindness, are at greater risk to be bullied or exposed to different traumatic experiences. Thus, the need for Theatre Practitioners to create more avenues where the Dramatic arts could be utilized in fostering healthy development and rehabilitation of at risk children becomes imperative.

The notion of Psychodrama, for example, is not a new concept in psychotherapy and indeed has been widely utilized in addressing psychosocial and learning weaknesses in at-risk children, adolescents and even adults. Developed by Romanian-American Psychiatrist, Jacob levy Moreno in 1910, Psychodrama explores the use of role playing and enactment of real life situations in an attempt to evaluate and redress the mental processes of the individual. This study proposes a critical analysis of the structures that make up the psycho-dramatic approach to child development as well as other related theories, putting into consideration the socio-economic conditions prevalent in the present African society.

In Nigeria, as well as in most African countries, scholars seem to agree that child development takes root from the indigenous or traditional education system that is inherent within the various socio-cultural enclaves of typical societies. This further implies that unifying structures of indigenous norms, practices and language are usually activated to solve communal issues. Mbachanga agrees when he observes that "Participatory performance on the one hand places priority on working with the people using their own mode of communication to enable small communities look at their own problems with the aim of arousing and stimulating target groups to take desired steps to improve their well-being" (87). The immediate society of a developing child plays a more important role than it is generally perceived to. Even with the influx of western education and its many inventions, African theorists seem to agree that the immediate surroundings of the child is more crucial in shaping his ideology towards life. The activities, therefore of his parents, relatives, teachers and other facilitators become an important ingredient in the development of a child. Ezenwa Ohaeto asserts that "The representation of childhood in African art, has to be approached from the standpoint that the African concept of childhood is profoundly different from that of childhood is profoundly different from that of the western world".

Children develop socially, intellectually, morally and psychologically and the cultural backgrounds of these children play significant roles in their development. As it concerns traditional education systems in Africa. Scholars seem to agree that activities and forms, such as imaginative play, begin from birth with the parents and other older relations playing the role of 'leader' or 'teacher-animator'. From this point, children through creative play, should develop socially and begin to develop their imaginative tendencies as can be expressed through role-playing where they take up roles like fathers, mothers, farmers or doctors. Other ideas could likewise be expressed through mime, music, dance and others. The daily events of children comprise of their relationship with people around their immediate environment such as their parents, friends and relatives. They meet people at home, at school or in places of worship and these relationships help to shape their ideology about themselves and their environment. Fayose P.O. believes that the ability for children to interact with others, enhances their relationship with members of their immediate society. He observes that "children's interpersonal relationship depend on their ability to express themselves through speech and movement".

In Nigeria for instance, research centered on Health humanities, with particular emphasis on children who could be suffering from Attention Deficit Hyperactive Disorder (ADHD) appear to be rather few. Some Nigerian scholars, who have ventured into this line of research, acknowledge that more attention should indeed be drawn to this area. Olusakin et al. note that "The lack of documented Nigeria-based research on ADHD makes this present work to be of relevance to Nigerians" (20). Some of the symptoms generally associated with children suffering from ADHD include, fidgeting with hands and feet, squirming in their seat, difficulty in sustaining attention and waiting for turn in tasks, games or group situations, difficulty in following through on instructions and experiences of a wide range in mood swings as well as having difficulty in delaying gratification.

Thus, where these traits are misconstrued as "spiritual problems", the child may be exposed to certain experiences that would further stunt positive development. Agazue Chima, in his review of Aaron Denham's book on the "Spirit Children of Northern Ghana", outlines that ethnographic pointers such as the historical, social, psychological, economic and political make up of these societies could be undeniable factors in the misconception of the children born in these localities. He observes that "The idea of the spirit child, according to Denham, "is intermeshed within *Nankani* material, relational and discursive worlds" (p.26). A spirit child "is not a human possessed by a spirit but rather is a simulacrum of a human, a spirit that only appears to be human" (p.92).The spirit children "are referred to as 'snakes' because many cannot walk; are perceived to be elusive, cunning and deceptive. And are as deadly as snakes" (pg70).They are often feared as spirits who took a human form with the intention of causing misfortune and destroying the family".

The use, thus of the rehabilitative capabilities of drama should not only ensure an improvement in social skills of developing children but should equip them in dealing with negative experiences that they may encounter. The study will evaluate four Applied Theatre projects across two states in Nigeria, in an attempt to properly underscore the impact of sustained theatrical activities to the plight of at-risk children and adolescents. The study engages the contribution of concepts such as Psychodrama and how the components of theatrical spontaneity and dramatic self-presentation can be brought to bear with the present realities of experiences relived by these members of the Nigerian society.

CHAPTER ONE

THE ISSUES CONFRONTING THE CHALLENGED CHILD IN NIGERIA

The term, 'Challenged Children', is used in this book to refer to children and adolescents who are unable to carry out optimal physical, mental and social activities and functions due to limitations ranging from medical conditions such as neurological and congenital deficiencies, to stunted psychosocial development as a result of debilitating environmental and communal practices and conjectures. Children may also become challenged from the impact of blunt force trauma caused by accidental mishaps, physical abuse and so on. The term specifically refers to the children within this study living with physical disabilities, visual impairment, Mental and Learning Challenges, Deafness, Dumbness, Down Syndrome, Albinism and so on.

Thus, the question of what should adequately be presented as an acceptable module for child learning, development and in peculiar cases, rehabilitation, is a major issue staring child educators and psychologists on their faces. There are individual, organisational and government efforts to formulate suitable child-development systems for the African child in general and the Nigerian child in particular. However, the extent to which these efforts provide for the needs of challenged children remains a thorny issue. Similarly, there is a persisting problem of the inadequate attention, the Nigerian educational system has given to at-risk children and their peculiar educational needs. According to the National Bureau of Statistics, Nigeria boasts of about 250 ethnic groups, with about 520 indigenous languages. While these appear to be advantageous in terms of rich cultural history and diversity, there are also challenges and differences along communal practices, belief systems, social values, as well as instructional and learning modules which have in turn put challenged children in more precarious situations.

A good child development system therefore, should prescribe for more effective methods of learning and indeed the reality that every child must pass through processes of birth, growth and development; scholars have put forward various suggestions on attitudinal as well as behavioral changes that could foster proper social responses from both healthy and challenged developing children. Indeed every research or inquiry should be geared towards answering given questions and proffering probable solutions to the problems plaguing society. Thus, the increasing cases of juvenile delinquency, child abuse, low self-esteem, bullying and drug abuse among challenged children and young adults should be given all the attention they deserve. Though the development needs of both normal and challenged children appeared minimal in the traditional society, with the wave of urbanization and population increase, their needs have trippled and made worse by ongoing redefinitions of the family support structure to accommodate new economic and technologically driven realities. Hence, some African scholars have continued to call for more parental and government involvement in the provision of educational aid, especially to the plight of challenged children, to forestall rising incidents of juvenile delinquency. There should also be a re-appreciation and integration of indigenous educational systems into new methods of child development. In affirmation of this position, Canice Nwosu queries "Prior to the enigmatic colonial encounter that ushered in African modernism; did the pre-colonial society experience Juvenile delinquency or militancy? One would say that the prevalent traditional socio-economic order equated with the type of disorder associated with the child then. There are strong indicators that sophistication in children and youth related crimes come with patterns in social and economic changes".

There are also other examples that put the average African child in an even more vulnerable conditions. The diverse religious, ethnic and cultural practices engaged in across the continent as well as high illiteracy levels appear to have created the misconception of certain traits that could rather be termed as socially influenced. These circumstances and others related to it are such that Art driven workshops could be utilized in creating new perceptions about how such problems could be tackled without adverse effects on the child and society.

The need to inject new approaches into the vast area of Applied Theatre Education and learning cannot be over emphasized. The myriad of concepts as brought forward by scholars may be suitable for certain situations and not for others. Thus, the need to adopt particular research strategies that would address issues of cognitive rehabilitation especially in at risk children and adolescents becomes imperative. Scholars have overtime acknowledged that children develop in stages and their perceptions, experiences and interpretation of the world is dependent on the stage in which they are. However, the questions of how they should be guided through the given stages and the preference for formal or informal education continue to raise the debate for the prerequisites for proper child development. David Pammenter observes that "The questions to be confronted are as stark now as they were 150 years ago, despite the tremendous steps forward during the intervening years. What is education? Who is it for, and what does it say we do? Is the school system the means by which we instills the inadequacies and contradictions of one social class or generation into the next? Or is it really concerned with freedom for children to develop their potential to the full; with equipping them to take an active part in shaping their world? Is it 'system-centered' or 'child-centered?".

CHAPTER TWO

THE ENGAGEMENT OF TRANSFORMATIVE LEARNING THEORIES IN REHABILITATIVE AND EDUCATIONAL EFFORTS

It would appear that the concept behind a transformative system of learning is one that does not view learning as a statutory and fixed exercise. Scholars have over time, formulated concepts on a variety of research enquires about ideal learning systems. Questions such as; who should learn? What should be learnt? How are learning environments created? What is expected in an appropriate teacher/learner relationship and how should the teacher/facilitator respond to certain needs of the learner, have contributed to the development of theories aimed at providing insight to the discourse of learning. "Learning theories have two chief values: one is in providing us with vocabulary and a conceptual framework for interpreting the examples of learning that we observe. The other is in suggesting where to look for solutions to practical problems" (Leonard, 17). This definition indicates that learning theories should create a spectrum for the analysis of certain variables rather than prescribe tailor-made solutions to learning needs. The thrust should be in bringing to the attention of researchers, knowledgeable facts and values needed for robust, indepth and analytical study on the subject of learning. Thus, some scholars have proposed that there exist three main conceptual frameworks where learning theories can be grouped. They are; Behaviorism, Cognitivism and Constructivism. The Behaviorist approach underscores those physical observable traits and aspects of Learning. Cognitivism evaluates the processes of psychologically induced learning and constructivism views learning from the process itself where new concepts and ideas are built upon.

"Transformative Learning is a deep, structural shift in basic premises of thought, feelings and action" (Transformative Learning Centre, 2004). Developed by American Sociologist, Jack Mezirow from 1978, The

Transformative learning theory was born out of the need to address, shifting behavioral patterns and thoughts due to internalized attitudes and perceptions. Orna Cohen et al, citing Mezirow submits that "Transformative learning refers to the process by which we transform our frames of reference to make them more inclusive, discriminating, open, emotionally capable of change and reflective so that they may generate beliefs and options that will prove true or justified to guide action".

One perspective to transformation, it would seem occurs in shared or personal experiences such as the death of a loved one, loss of a job, the occurrence of a natural disaster and so on. These experiences may cause individuals to question hitherto held beliefs and even the essence of their existence. Edward Taylor observes that "learning experiences establish a common base from which each learner constructs meaning through personal reflections and group discussion" (6). Mezirow's Transformative learning theory has evolved into a comprehensive and complex description of how learners interpret and validate the meaning of their experience. Mezirow identifies ten phases for transformative learning which is a process of how given perspectives and structural meaning are changed or revised. These phases develop from feelings of disorienting dilemma, guilt or shame to critical assessments of social-cultural or psychic assumptions and then exploring new relationships and actions which ultimately should increase individual confidence and competence levels within these new roles. (Kitchenham, 105)

Recent studies however hold that these phases could be grouped into four elaborate broader steps for a better understanding of the prospective for transformation and more workable results. Orna Cohen et al submits that "These steps include experiencing a disorienting dilemma where the learner struggles with a conflict of views, because a current understanding of their frame of reference doesn't fit anymore. This leads to imitation or confusion, because meaningful solution cannot be found immediately to critically assessing assumptions such that the frame of reference is questioned. The learner is going through self-examination, assessing previously held assumptions to find ways out of the dilemma. The learner also acquires and implements while observing other people's reactions and behaviors; a rational dialogue evolves and he discovers new information, which is put into perspective with the old assumptions. And then the final stage where he or she explores options for new roles, relationship and actions: The learner practices the newly acquired skills and knowledge, finding new roles and competences.

A new self- confidence evolves and new relationships build. As a result, the learner replaces "old views" and gains a new perspective".

Scholars have argued that for a broader understanding of the transformative learning theory to be acquired, certain perspectives must be underscored to give credence to the research works being carried out in this area. These perspectives should be such that integrates psycho-analytic views such as the learning process of the individual; the state of understanding oneself, one's inner identity, persona, confidence, self empowerment and responsibility. A psycho-developmental perspective is also critical in understanding the demand aspects of continuous, incremental and progressive growth as well as the appreciation for behavioral differences and the role of relationships.

A social-emancipatory perspective is also crucial in giving consideration to the role of social change in the transformative learning process. Scholars like Edward W. Taylor propose that the social-emancipatory perspective of Transformative learning gives a certain level of responsibility to the society in addressing concerns faced by its individuals. Rooted primarily in the Freirean concept of *Conscientization*, which views people as subjects not objects, constantly reflecting on the transformation of their world, Taylor believes that the goal of social transformation could be enhanced by "demythicizing reality"(8)., thereby allowing the oppressed to develop a sense of critical consciousness. This process should not only engender critical reflection and engage dialogical methodologies but must also adopt a horizontal learner/teacher relationship to stimulate a participatory learning process. He observes that: "Three teaching approaches are central to fostering emancipatory transformative learning. First is the centrality of critical reflection, with the purpose of rediscovering power and helping learners develop an awareness of agency to transform society and their own reality. Second, a liberating approach to teaching couched in "acts of cognition, not in transferal of information". It is a problem posing and dialogical methodology. Third is a horizontal students-teacher relationship where the teacher works as a political agent and on an equal footing with student".

Thus, the role of society and indeed the teacher in this context forms an important factor in Transformative learning. The Freireian and likeminded schools of thought propose that teachers should educate for transformation; the Teacher should be adequately prepared to work through concerns and challenges the learning process may present and this includes creating new avenues where knowledge is not only built upon but co-created by the students. Citing Bailey on the intellectual partnership between mentors and mentees through the lens of the Transformative learning theory, Margareth S. Zanchetta et al submit that "Intellectual partnerships are built on the beliefs and intentions of social transformation and personal empowerment of student and teachers. From the standpoint of constructivism, this transformation is attained through the facilitation of different ways of thinking and formulating answers. In intellectual partnerships, teachers are able to identify and learn new ways to foster students' education by building on their ideas and facilitating co-creation of knowledge. Students are able to participate in the production of knowledge and pursue their goals in various contexts".

However, there are other views which propose a slight departure from the constructivist approach to transformative learning. Further researches indicate that for transformation to occur, learning must progress beyond building on existing knowledge. Scholars like Janik, D. and Edward Taylor observe that neurobiological and cultural components are emerging in the field of transformation learning and that these components, when integrated into the process engenders learning that is 'brain based' and discovery driven. In this context the teacher/facilitator plays a supervisory and assisting role more effectively. Janik posits that "In simpler terms, the findings suggest that the brain structure usually changes during the learning process. These findings in turn bring into question traditional models of learning (behaviourism congitivism, Constructivism) and instead offer a distinctive neurobiological, physically based pathway to transformative learning. From this perspective, learning is seen as "volitional, curiosity based, discovery-driven and mentor-assisted" and most effective at higher cognitive levels".

The introduction of Transformative learning in children poses a unique challenge for teachers and facilitators. The need to equip the developing child in facing the demands of society becomes imperative especially when certain present conditions appear to stunt the development process. Within African and indeed Nigeria, present economic realities indicate that today's growing child is currently faced with developmental needs that are crucial for holistic psychosocial growth and well being. The Nigeria Bureau of statistics reports that as at 2016, about 76% percent of Nigeria's population live below the poverty line. The Brooklyn's institution Report cited in Emmanuel Okogba's article on "Nigeria's deepening poverty misery" in the Vanguard issue of 2nd July, 2018, reveals that "at the end of may 2018, our trajectories support that

Nigeria had about 87 million people in extreme poverty compared with India's 73 million, Nigeria has overtaken India as the country with the largest number of extreme poor" (n.pag). This economic reality however is most likely to spiral down other social structures thereby causing corresponding increase in loss of jobs, disease outbreaks, broken marriages, deaths and so on. In these situations, the vulnerability of the growing child increases the tendency for him to become a causality of circumstance.

Transformative learning thus, should provide Educative and Rehabilitative institutions, the potential to equip the child adequately for present and possible future challenges. The child should not just be an active participant in the learning process, but should be able to ask vital questions on what he has learnt, what he is being taught and how all these can help him formulate his own perceptions about his existence and his environment. Mezirow and Kitchenham cited by Zanchetta *et'al* submit that "The theory emphasizes principles that foster the development of critical consciousness, political liberation and awareness, beyond the usual outcomes of traditional teaching. The purpose of learning should be to develop autonomous, empowered thinkers, who are able to adopt to change, think critically and take action to change their lives by critically examining their experiences".

Indeed the child-learner should be encouraged through activities that will propel development. This can be through exercises that will not only sustain their interest but enable them confront given problems and proffer solutions to them. Children appear to enjoy learning where there is an attempt to make the process enthusiastic and lively. However, since a greater part of their thinking is still tied to what is seen and heard, the teacher/facilitator is challenged to employ deft skill within the educative endeavour to sustain their interest in the creative process. The Transformative learning theory in this context provides for learning that is both task-oriented and communicative. The essence is to allow for the learners to engage themselves constructively in the learning process as supervised by the teacher/facilitators while being able to communicate their feelings and needs. Scholars prescribe that for a holistic learning process to be achieved there should exist a detailed application of curricular content so as to ensure that the performance of the learners is appropriately evaluated. Richard Cullata posits that "Applying transformative theory to curriculum evaluation, one looks for evidence of critical reflection in terms of content, process and premise. Content reflection consists of curriculum mapping from students and faculty perspective; process reflection focuses best practices, literature-based indicators and self efficacy measures; premise reflection would consider both content and process reflection to develop recommendations".

Transformative learning with the aid of Drama and theatrical or performative activities appear to have a stake in child learning and development. The ability to utilize drama in mirroring society places the Theatre on a uniquely distinct plane in addressing issues of individual and social transformation. Drama allows us to understand the complexities of human behaviour; Relatively, Transformative learning as E.O. Sullivan observes "involves experiencing a shift, such a shift involves our understanding of ourselves, our location, our relationship with other humans and the natural world" (4). Indeed, scholars have proposed that educative processes even in the context of formal learning can be further enhanced with the integration of creative, dramatic activities. This has given rise to concepts such as Theatre in Education (TiE), Creative Dramatics, Drama in Education, Applied Theatre, Play-House Theatre and many others which among other things, propose for an engaging participatory frontier to learning in order to foster, creativity, spontaneity, ingenuity and propel positive social responses to the process of learning and development. Chiduo Obadiegwu further corroborates this, indicating that the qualitative research designs would be adequate in evaluating the level of participation in this area of study. He affirms that, "Since theatre education for transformative learning focuses on participation and exploration of voices of the learners, qualitative research designs is appropriate for children's real participation in the classroom".

Theatre scholars seem to agree that concepts of drama within educational systems are capable of stimulating positive responses to learning challenges. Through creative play, children develop socially and begin to explore their imaginative tendencies on addressing simulated problems, institutions of learning provide. Drama achieves this through exercises of role playing and interpretation, thematic construction and so on. Fayose opines that "drama tells a story through actions and because the issues connected with the story are acted out by human beings, the message is brought more realistically home to the reader or viewer".

Transformative learning thus, through drama could serve as an indispensable tool in facilitating the development of thinking and language skills in children. Through positive metacognitive development, children master rules for directing their own attention, thoughts and behaviour thereby fostering positive forms of expression.

Transformative Aspects in Art Therapy and the Psychodrama Approach

A number of concepts appear to find expression on the therapeutic components of Art. Scholars have argued that Art; be it visual or performative possesses strong potential in causing positive psychological and behavioral change. Interventions such as the Cognitive Behavioral Art Therapy (CBAT), which combines cognitive and behavioral therapies like cognitive restructuring, breathing exercises and psycho-education with Artistic expressions like paintings and sculptures, have recorded successes in aiding persons with anxiety issues or other psychological disorders.

On a study on the integration of Art into Cognitive behavioral Therapy for anxiety disorders such as the Panic Disorder with Agoraphobia (PDA) and Generalized Anxiety Disorder (GAD), Francis J. Morris reports that in case 1 for PDA, "The intervention resulted in statistically significant reductions in Panic frequency and some features of Panic anxiety and agoraphobia. In case 2 for GAD, the decrease in general anxiety was marginally significant" (343). Indeed, as a necessitated improvement on the cognitive behavioural therapy (CBT), the CBAT incorporates the role of Art in fostering deeper levels of focus and commitment to the behavioural restructuring process. Morris, informs that "CBT requires clients to think abstractly for a variety of tasks, including visualization and ranking exercises. These exercises may be challenging for some clients with lower verbal skills or more concrete thinking".

However, the integration of Art therapy allows for the participants or clients in this case to be more actively engaged in the process of their transformation, rather than merely being 'spoon fed' by the therapists. Acknowledging studies carried out by scholars like Curry and Kasser (2005), Chambak (2008), Sandmire et al (2012) and Vander Vennet and serice (2012), Morris, observes that "Art therapy, including Mandalas, collage, drawing, painting and sculpting, significantly reduced state and trait anxiety over control groups in college students prior to final examinations. Art therapists commonly employ the process of drawing or coloring mandalas-circular, geometric pattern to focus or relax clients. Curry and Kasser (2005), also found the colouring of mandalas and other geometric patterns significantly reduced anxiety in college students. The complex structure of the design encouraged a meditative state while reducing extraneous thinking. Van *der* Vennet and Serice (2012) replicated this study with similar findings".

The performative aspect and quality of Art may be viewed as an equally effective intervention for Therapy and Rehabilitation. Indeed, studies show that the performing Arts either in the context of Dance or Drama possess far reaching potentials in engendering psycho-social and behavioral change. The concept of Dance/movement therapy for instance, emerged around 1950 in North America as an interdisciplinary field, composed of the creative and expressive characteristics of dance as well as knowledge and methods in psychotherapy (Chin Lee, 400). Thus, as an Art form, Dance involves bodily movements and expressions that are capable of stimulating feelings and thoughts in an individual as well as inducing communicative expressions with the world around him.

Scholars and Dance therapists such as Tsung Chin Lee argue that as an integrative discipline, Dance and movement therapy is intricately subsumed in the language and expressions of the body rather than the sole focus of verbal communication. In a study carried out by Chin Lee on the impact of Dance/movement therapy on psychiatric patients with depression, she underscores Schmais (1974) and Dosamantes-Alperson, (1981) when she submits that "Movement serve as an intermediary between the inner and outer world, whereby a patient may be able to truly contact his/her psyche and thus, enable the function of self healing. In the therapeutic process, one's feeling/thoughts may be transformed through the moving body and in turn, the bodily expression of the feelings/thoughts, changes".

She further observes that "Movements activate an interactive process between one's outward expression and inner feelings/thoughts, and serve as a gateway between one's inner and outer world. Through expressive movements, one becomes aware of oneself and opens the self to the outer world. The perception of one's self in relation to the outer world keeps unfolding throughout one's own movement to movement and unique experience in the body: that is, the process of one's change is somehow corporal and differs from person to person".

Thus, Dance which makes very elaborate use of bodily movements, integrates other factors such as perception, imagination and feeling in a fluid concept such that within the construct of behavioural and psychological rehabilitation, each factor may not be estranged from the other. In the course of research, for instance, Chin Lee evaluates the application of dance therapy to the case of a middle-age Taiwanese woman, appropriately given the pseudonym (Chun-Li) and diagnosed with major depression with psychotic features. In the course of the therapy, Lee ascertained that traumatic and experiences borne out of a psychologically intolerable and abusive marriage were factors in the decline of Chun Li's health for which she had been hospitalized up to three times for spells of two to three months. With the gradual introduction of Ballroom, Qi Gong and flying dance routines, Chun Li eventually learns to cope with the feelings of loss and conflict in a much healthier way. Tsung-Chin Lee reports that "Her body was induced by the virtual ardent look to express allure and then, with the prolonged repetition of her imagination over time, to invariably perform the allure increasingly, intensely in order to attract more and more appreciation and looks. In reverse, the charming swings and graceful gestures increased her happiness and originated other sensory experiences and movements".

Drama therapy, which is also a performative process, can be utilized in improving psychological skills in children and Adults alike. Indeed, Drama therapy can be defined as the systematic and intentional use of drama/theatre to achieve psychological change and growth. (Emunah, 1994). Scholars inform that other manifestations of Drama therapy include Psychodrama, Playback theatre, Movement drama and so on which basically acknowledges the relevance as well as interdependence of health and creativity in an approach that cuts across disciplines. Dayton cited in Butler et al, (2013) states that "drama therapy allows for a creative symbolic expression of thinking, feeling and behaviour that can lead to an enhanced creativity and spontaneity in the individual and an increased ability to perceive and take action toward desirable life choices".

The similarity of the art forms of dance and drama in the context of therapy perhaps lies in the activity and conscious involvement of thoughts and body movements to create healthy energy where psychological development could thrive. It has been observed that movement can be used to communicate. Thus, the ability not just to understand the meaning of bodily expressions as can be espoused through drama or dance, but also to channel these art forms as therapeutic media becomes imperative in inducing positive behavioural and psychological development in dealing with children or adolescents. The drama-therapist could employ deft skill in a group setting, where the participants are assisted to resolve problems through creative ways. This in turn creates an environment, for example, through the instrumentality of drama, where the voices, stories, bodies and reflections of the participants and the group in general, play an important role in improving teacher-participant relations and inadvertently increasing the therapeutic potential of the process. Butler et al maintains that "Therapeutic change occurs through an intricate interplay of various guided human experiences. The therapy analogue of the client-therapist relationship becomes broader in group therapy. Every participant in psychodrama is a potential therapeutic agent to the others. It is therefore important to organize a therapeutic drama group in such a way that a therapeutic atmosphere can develop and cohesiveness can be established".

In a ten-week South African Project, Elmien Butler, Terri M. Bakker and Gerhard Viljoen report on the use of "movement drama" as a therapeutic approach of drama in transforming language and fostering more responsive and poetic ways of dealing with problems as well as exploring new ways of thinking. In the workshop, 13 adolescents between the ages of 13 and 17 were selected into a group. Even though the composition of the group appeared skewed because all the participants had interests in drama as a medium of expression, the researchers regarded the project as a success as there were evident and recorded progress in creative imagination expression and a better awareness of self. The project reports that "Group therapy criteria were taken into consideration as the author planned the group meetings and process. In the end, the participants who took part in the research project, met on a weekly basis for 90min for 10 weeks. The session took place in a large multipurpose room with chairs, drama blocks, a sound system and some props. The author wanted to use the metaphor of the director rehearsing with a group of actors and an unknown script. The performative and creative process created a therapeutic community of discovery and growth that were observed and explored as part of the research project".

The Movement drama concept, thus as an offshoot of Psychodrama and Drama therapy presents as a participant-based dramatic workshop where different units of certain themes and phenomena are analyzed through creative exercises that stimulate self exploration, narration, ingenuity and group work. These exercises, scholars observe should be chosen specifically to suit the particular need of the group as well as incite the participants to express themselves openly and directly while creating a feeling of comfort and shared interest, giving them the opportunity to explore their minds and bodies in creative, therapeutic and dramatic ways (Butler, 2013). The end result among others should include a development of the concept of the body as a symbol of empowerment as well as a broader understanding of the narrative essence of drama, as expressed through activities like storytelling, in expanding the therapeutic space and motivating the possibilities of creating better alternative stories and self descriptions. Reporting on the efficacy of the South African drama therapy project, Butler et al state that "In a follow-up group interview of 90mins, 1 month after the performance, the adolescents reported a deeper awareness of self and others as well as experiences related to personality integration and enhanced relationships. The interview data were recorded on DVD, and findings were summarized from studying the material. Their talk reflected a sense of empowerment through creating a harmonious language between minds and bodies".

The Psychodramatic approach to character modeling and psychological development follow similar patterns and mediums albeit differences in structure and execution. The development of psychodrama by Jacob Levy Moreno in 1910 was also borne out of the necessity to improve cognitive and behavioral exploration, engender healthy emotional responses and insight as well as induce therapeutic change in significant areas of human life. It is primarily utilized as an action method which engages spontaneous dramatization through role playing and dramatic self presentation in enacting real life situations on stage. Scholars and therapists alike have argued that the integration of psychodrama in rehabilitating 'at risk' children and adolescents should not only improve the client-therapist therapeutic bond but should also increase client dramatic engagement and involvement in the process significantly. However, there are certain differences in the approaches of psychodrama and Drama therapy. Whereas both psychodrama and drama therapy use dramatic techniques and processes for therapeutic change, Orkibi et al observe that "Clinically, in psychodrama clients typically use role-play to enact themselves, parts of themselves or significant others in their real lives and hence work more directly on their issues. In contrast, drama therapy is more fantasy-based and clients typically use role-play to enact fictional and symbolic roles, engage in storytelling, puppetry and rituals to work more indirectly and with greater distance from their issues".

Some scholars and practitioners have maintained that psychodrama should be executed and is effective from within a group. Indeed, participants may draw connections to their own circumstances from the enactment of another's. In practice, a protagonist is chosen at each given time whose issues represent the main elements of the group. Societal issues such as stigma, unacceptance, racial discrimination etc can be bought forward thus instigating more scenes accordingly. These scenes are enacted and repeated not just to recreate societal responses, but to educate the group on the proper responses to the same issues. Recent studies on psychodrama and its impact on children and Adolescents seem to indicate an increase in dramatic engagement of the participants covered as well as improved productive behaviours. An understudy of research enquiries from Shechtman and Katz (2007), Leichtentritt and Shechtman (2010)., by Hod, Orkibi et al reveal that "In a study on Israel adolescents, bonding with the therapist contributed to out comes more than bonding with group members. In another study, higher scores on bonding predicted decreased anxiety and aggression as well as increased social competence. In a study on group art therapy, bonding as reported by both child and therapist predicted decreases in child-reported internalizing and externalizing behavioral symptoms".

In related studies, psychodrama has been utilized in building healthy interpersonal relationships and evaluating attachment concepts in young adults with a view to investigate the differences between healthy emotional relationship and psychological health. Developed by making use of the Theatre of spontaneity, Psychodrama appears to offer additional benefits other than those already known. Through the enactment of past experiences, psychodrama participants gain insight into the mental representations they have developed through the relationships they have encountered and are presently encountering. By doing so, individuals with insecure attachment values recognize the impact of these values on their relationships and alter them where necessary. Furthermore, participants may through psychodrama gain behavioural and emotional insight into their situation at the time and improve both social and empathy skills. Turkan Dogan observes that "Participants in a self-development psychotherapy group use feedback from others and self observation to realize the important aspects, strengths and boundaries of their own interpersonal behaviours, their interpersonal conflicts and their maladaptive behaviours that attract negative reactions from others. Participants not only become aware of their personal responsibility in the shaping of interpersonal relationships but also realize their power to change them. As a method of psychotherapeutic and socio-therapeutic action, psychodrama is a particular life like form of group psychotherapy".

Moreno defines psychodrama as an approach which studies the existence of humanity and the realities in different life situations by using dramatic methods. Psychodrama gives individuals a chance to enact their problems rather than only talk about them (Dogan, 113). Thus, the experiences enacted in psychodrama allow participants to rehearse more ideal future circumstances while helping them live through present experiences and situations. Through the concept of realistic enactment, traumatic situations are recreated as they were in the past, however, with the re-enactment, the participants are better equipped to deal with the situation. Indeed, as Moreno cited in Dogan (2010) states, "every second experience liberates people from the first. In psychodrama, past events, future hopes and fears are transmitted to present time and resolved"

Psychodrama as a form of psychotherapy has been viewed to be quite instructive in dealing with traumatic and anxiety-related circumstances. In 2013, a study was carried out in Merano, Italy on five secondary school students who had increased anxiety levels on the subject of mathematics. Psychodrama was introduced as a new intervention in the relatively unresearched area. Gsterin Dorothea informs that "Research on different forms of therapy and their specific interventions, which are apt to alleviate pupils' and students' anxiety related to mathematics, are practically inexistent. Currently there are no studies that show the effectiveness of psychodrama as a treatment for adolescents who suffer from mathematics anxiety. This study can therefore be considered a first attempt to bring some light into a completely dark and unexplored area of research".

The concept, thus of utilizing the psychodramatic approach in dealing with anxiety-related circumstances perhaps stems from Moreno's view of Anxiety as being opposed to the element of spontaneity which is a vital component in psychodrama. Moreno's ideology establishes anxiety and spontaneity at opposite sides of psychological development, and that anxiety sets in because spontaneity is absent. Thus the restraint of spontaneity which the avenue of Drama provides stifles creativity, and limits the choices of the individual. Whereas, anxiety increases a state of dormancy and robotic disposition to situations. The study carried out by Gstrein indicated that pupils and students suffering mathematics anxiety definitely lack spontaneity and experience limited choices of reactions. Especially before and in test situations, when their worrisome thoughts grow out of proportion; they are locked at one and of the continuum, at the anxiety end (201). Further observations reveal that "The most frequently mentioned problems regarded their nervousness before a math test, their increased stress level, their inability to concentrate during the test, as well as continuous defeatist self talk. Some pupils reported somatic disorders, stomach ache or headache or sleep disorders before a math test. All of the pupils interviewed said that their motivation to learn mathematics was rather low, that they often compared their performances with schoolmates and that their perceived self-efficacy related to mathematics was extremely low".

In other seemingly traumatic or potentially traumatic situations, scholars have proposed that psychodrama as well as other psychodramatic derivations of Drama therapy such as the concept of 'Play back' Theatre could be potentially effective in dealing with situations ranging from unhealthy and toxic relationships to identity crisis management. The ability to foster a deeper awareness of self as well as develop healthy relationships that are crucial for social and psychological development is vital to the integration of psychodrama. Evaluating a Korean study on the subject, Soo Eun Chae et al submit that "Psychodrama can be useful in enhancing the adjustment, development, and interpersonal relationships of college students who face various psychological challenges and of time, crises. Psychodrama can be particularly beneficial to Korean college students who engrain themselves in habitual patterns due to the restrictions placed upon them by the collectivist culture valuing face and appearance, and revealing themselves as they really are".

A 12-session psychodrama workshop carried out in Ankara, Turkey, with 21 masters level students participating and extending over 3 months, evaluated the concept of the understanding of self as well as coping with and developing the sense of self confidence, self worth and empathy. The participant feedback of the experimental group revealed the following in the Chart below:

Participant	**Feedback about gains**
Participant 1 (female)	Recognizing that the problems they encounter in their relationships are similar to those of other participants and relaxing: getting rid of feelings of Isolation.
Participant 2 (male)	Accepting that it is natural to experience problems: approaching people more comfortably.
Participant 3 (female)	Improvement in empathy skills: feeling more positive and light: coping with being hurt: looking forward instead of back.
Participant 4 (male)	Eliminating selfishness in relationships: listening more, sharing and making sacrifices: overcoming moodiness and improvement in logical thinking.
Participant 5 (female)	Letting go of ex-relationships: stop making excuses and seeing emotions and events more objectively: recognizing one's capacity of coping and that problems are natural.

Participant 6 (female)	Finding comfort in the fact that others have similar problems and finding novel solutions.
Participant 7 (female)	Noticing that a positive outlook is important accepting rather than judging: understanding that she is in control of a relationship and becoming aware of one's inner power.
Participant 8 (female)	Starting to look around and open oneself more: being more open in romantic relationships: seeing that others have similar problems and having a more positive outlook on life.
Participant 9 (female)	Improvement in understanding males: gaining experience.
Participant 10 (female)	Recognizing when a partner does not value his/her feelings: having more self-confidence in Romantic relationships. (Dogan, 116)

Turkan, Dogan further informs that: "The qualitative data of the study revealed an improvement in participants' empathy skills and awareness of attachment styles too. For instance, in the "decision making in a nuclear family" group play in the third session, a female participant who played the role of a "father who is cheating on his wife" managed to establish empathy with her own father as a result of this role, and developed insight into her lack of trust for the opposite sex and the reasons why she is afraid of being hurt".

Indeed, the numerous examples of traumatic experiences around the world have invariably increased the cases of stigmatized individuals. Children who fall within a category that can at best be termed as vulnerable are at greater risk of being stigmatized especially where other factors, not favourable to positive development, are present. A number of studies indicate that mental disorders in growing children and adults alike may likely find firmer footing in stigma-induced environments. However, theatre methods have been used as instruments to promote inclusion of mental health patients in local communities; the performance-making process has proved to reduce prejudice and discrimination, promote health and build social networks (Bosco et al 2014). Derivatives from the psychodramatic approach such as the playback theatre engages these methods in promoting community education as well as engendering positive social and behavioural change in individuals with psychosocial needs. Yotis et al submit that "Transformative experiences of patients with schizophrenia during performance-making related to the safety of the therapeutic structure, role-playing and formation of connections, help to overcome the challenges of dysfunction and achieve a sense of well being. Playback Theatre has been reported to promote mental health, creating a journey towards a valued sense of identity, role and purpose beyond the diagnosis of mental illness".

However, it is critical to note that in the different psychodrama projects carried out, scholars also indicate that the approach does not guarantee a rubber-stamped recipe for success whenever utilized. Indeed, emphasis is dwelt on the process as well as each experience derived from a given study. As Blatner cited in Dan Yaniv (2011) observes that "They are five basic constituents of psychodrama: the protagonist is the person who represents the themes of the group drama and whose experience is the primary focus of the drama, auxiliary egos are represented by group members who assume the roles of significant others in the protagonist's drama; the audience are those group members who witness the drama and represent the world at large, and the director is a trained psychodramatist who guides participants through each phase of the session and is responsible for the therapeutic process".

The aforementioned process guides the primary concept of psychodrama and indeed other forms of Drama therapy. Even though psychodramatic approaches have been integrated into different spheres of psychotherapy, it is probable that a number of factors could increase or decrease the level of progress. On the effectiveness of psychodrama on Mathematics anxiety, Gstrein Dorothea reports her findings; stating that "Regarding motivation to learn mathematics only one student convincingly declared that this goal had been reached. None of the participants said that the psychodrama training had fundamentally changed their motivation to study mathematics, however all the students reported that some changes in their attitude towards mathematics had occurred".

The report given by Turkan Dogan on the Ankara Psychodrama workshop, similarly observed that "the quantitative findings of the study showed that the psychodrama group helped lower participants' anxiety levels. At the same time, no meaningful difference was observed between the experimental and control groups on the anxiety dimension".

The British Association of Dramatherapists as cited by Susan Cassidy, define Drama therapy as "the intentional use of healing aspects of drama and Theatre as a therapeutic process. It is a method of working and playing that uses action methods to facilitate creativity, imagination, learning and growth". The North American Drama Therapy Association agrees, defining it as "An active, experiential approach to facilitating change, through storytelling, projective play, purposeful improvisation and performance; Participants are invited to rehearse desired behaviors, expand and find flexibility between life roles and perform the change they wish to be and see in the world".

Drama therapy and attendant approaches such as psychodrama primarily rely on descriptive, theoretical, clinical and creative work that are significant in identifying integrating and analyzing methods that are effective in creating desired changes in participants with regard to psychological health and the ability to utilize Theatre in dealing with forms of Trauma, Jacques Arpin asks these questions "What can a healer learn from Theatre and performance studies? What can Theatre and performance studies bring to healing practices? Both disciplines are distinct in Western societies; at times merge into miscellaneous forms of "art therapy". What lessons can we learn from traditions that do not separate these competencies and have always integrated them as being naturally complementary?"

The different misconceptions about how young persons who live with varied degrees of physical or mental challenges are perceived and/or understood were also observed to have given rise to ideological conflicts as well as social attitudes and practices. Theatre thus was utilized in bringing the practices to the fore using the immediacy, the dramatic medium provides in activating needed interactions, conversations and mobilized action on issues ranging from Abuse, depression, bullying to lack of adequate care and misconstrued communal practices.

Findings of the study propose an increase in psychosocial awareness and development as well as improved levels of cognitive activities in challenged children and adolescents with the sustained introduction of dramatic activities; such that is both participatory in nature yet tailored to address distinct social and environmental constructs as well as individual challenges encountered by the participants. Indeed, in more recent times, there appears to be an increase in the engagement of multi-disciplinary approaches especially in education as well as in health care delivery and practice. The application of drama in addressing learning challenges and needs in children continues to be explored as an interventionist approach capable of engendering qualitative transformation and development. In Nigeria more scholars are beginning to propose for the integration of performance based activities in the development of imaginative and verbal skills required for holistic child education. In

Obadiegwu's words "Here lies the relationship between drama and education because drama encourages the development of individual personal resources. These resources are the sensory perception, intellect, imagination, power of concentration, physical and verbal skill and emotional control. All these are essential for the child's development and drama is one of the means of harmonizing them for the benefits of the growing child".

Further studies, thus propose that the therapeutic integration of Drama should create an environment where positive development is not only possible but should thrive. The contribution of the dramatic Arts to society, which has also found expression in the social and Health sciences allows for a recreation of society as it is and as it should be, such that participants in the creative process and the society at large engage more in fostering new ways that are ideal for holistic development.

CHAPTER 3

ORAL TRADITIONS IN AFRICA AS A COMPONENT IN THE REHABDRAMATICS APPROACH

In most African countries, Nigeria inclusive, scholars have maintained that there is indeed need to reintegrate proper value systems as emanating from indigenous and tradition norms and culture into the sphere of daily co-existence. For these theorists, Africa's rich cultural practices and norms provide balanced remedies for the variety of life's experiences and challenges. Indeed, some scholars have argued that the ideology of Globalization as given accentuation by the imperialist stance of western influence may have had adverse effects on the development of the continent. It is proposed that indigenous, cultural norms and practices which includes oral and performative literature and enactments, possess instructive elements in engaging present discourses and phenomena such as social injustice, governance, parenthood, child development and so on. Ezenweke observes that "Africa has rich cultural values, coated with sense of sacredness which aided African civilization and which seemed to have been swept off by the wind of globalization. This has hitherto, affected life in many African societies in general, Nigeria in particular".

The scholars support that rather than solve problems emanating from the communicative needs of individuals, the concept of globalization may have even created some of its own and by so doing, have affected the scared fabric of communal interaction and living. Odimegwu avers that, 'with the use of technology like satellite radio and television, the phones, the traditional concepts and notions of space, time and distance have been drastically affected, reduced and redefined' (23). Thus, it is viewed that the influx of globalization into various African societies may have introduced isolationist approaches to social relations which negate the communal nature ofbrotherhood, collectivism and an appreciation of human worth and equality in the African community. The oral and performative aspects of traditional and cultural practices in

Africa appear laden with instructive material that can engender psychosocial interaction as well as development in individuals. The utilization of the Folk media, for instance, as expressed through forms such as folksongs, folklore, folkgames, dances, puppetry, proverbs, and so on, employ very descriptive and in some cases, reformative approaches in engaging the imaginative and conscious abilities of the individual to real situations and issues. Williams Onogu states that "In the context of using folk media, for development communication, emphasis is on development of the psychological, intellectual and physical resources of the individual which is aimed at self-initiative. Art forms of expression such as folktales, folk-dances, folk music, proverbs, etc are available folk media aspects for rural communication in development".

The integration of indigenous art forms such as the folk media into Applied Theatre workshops like Theatre for Development (TfD) and Theatre in Education (TiE), allows for an incorporation of these art forms that would engender development. Onogu observes that "folk musicians and singers serve as social critics, educators and development activists towards oppression, injustice, exploitation etc. Emuejevoke Omoko speaks of the Urhobo popular songs tradition as "An indigenous oral poetic tradition that is composed and performed by singers who celebrate the exploits and qualities of individuals, groups, animal characters and things. They also comment on social and existential matters in order to influence public morality. The popular songs tradition relies on eulogizing those aspects or norms of society that others should emulate for the general good of society".

The folkloric tradition appears equally effective in driving needed points on societal issues. The infusion of proverbs and poetic sayings enlarges the descriptive material while inducing reflective thinking. On the relevance of proverbs in the context of oral tradition in Africa, Yusuf cited by Ekegbo et al state that "Proverbs as we know, form a vital sector of folklore which has survived centuries of impartial relegation of African cultural legacies and heritage. Proverbs are rhetorical devices which enhance the ability of the speaker to make a speech in a concise, figurative and enriched manner, far in advance of what plan and ordinary speech can do".

The effectiveness of Africa's oral literary tradition perhaps lies in its potential as an educative medium as well as its use as a mechanism in addressing social character. This is more efficient and expressive with the integration of a people's own art forms and culture within the concientization process. Muleka, Joseph states that, "the question of what constitutes oral literature is a complex one. It perhaps calls for a very clear understanding of the principles that govern the people's appreciation of their own creative verbal art"87. Indeed, on the concept of child-centered development, scholars propose that the African oral tradition provide a very expressive environment for the child. Art forms such as folk songs, folk lore, games, chants and dances provide moral, cultural and even historical perspectives about life, the activities of folk lore and songs for example, appeals to the imagination of the child and as such engender not just physical participation but psychological participation as well. The essence of holistic participation is key to the development process of child. Ray Emeana as cited by Arinze-Umobi on the process of the story telling culture in Africa observes that "During moonlight entertainment, the mother, father, grandfather or indeed any of the children would lead the story session depending on the circumstances. Most of the tales are structured in such a manner as to allow the audience to fully participate in the chants, music and dance, while the narrator moves around directing the narration to the audience as the characters in the story may demand".

The concept of participation here, presupposes that the collective effort of every member of society is a crucial determinant in achieving child-centered development. In instances where the child is placed as at-risk either due to genetic or environmental anomalies, the society's response and action, provides as a basis for holistic development. Some of these art forms may be utilized in addressing a variety of themes such as Hardwork, Respect, ill-treatment of others and so on. These examples thus possess unique traits in conveying deep meanings that could be instrumental in causing changes in thought processes and social attitudes.

Augusto Boal's conception of the Theatre for the oppressed feeds into this narrative on the critical importance for participants or in this, community members in African societies to take necessary action on issues that affect their own lives; Thus, the coinage of the term 'Spec-actors', which thrusts members of the audience into the action-taking process. A matrix of Boal's dramatic techniques and Paulo Freire's democratic principles of group inquiry and the community-based science paradigm inform commitment of research and advocacy efforts to partnerships that investigate root causes as well as addressing health and social outcomes of environmental injustices".

The instrumentality of the Theatre, thus allows for a creative process that is participatory so as to engender communal input in the change effort. The effort culminates in a workshop laced with physical games, character creation and image-making exercises, improvisation and even scene construction. Boal outlines the process thus "Knowing the body- exploring limitations, balance, improvisational possibilities and social distortions. Making the body expressive- dehabituation, learning vocabulary and syntax of dramatic physicality. Theatre as language- simultaneous dramaturgy, image theatre and the forum. Theatre as discourse- thematic spectacles".

Indeed, Scholars seem to agree that the integration of concepts such as the Theatre of the oppressed provides for the application and engagement of community-based methodology in engendering investigative and collaborative intervention where facilitators work in tandem with the community to understand and resolve community problems and also to democratize this participatory process so as to adequately empower members of community. The community-Based participatory Research (CBPR), for instance acknowledges acquisition in the development process knowledge as viewed as an instrument of power and control and this begs the need for a leveraging and channeling of this factor in order to decentralize the power dynamic to foster inclusiveness. In the same vein, Justice Sullivan et al reiterates "Defined as a collaborative approach to research that equitably involves all partners in the research process and recognises the unique strength that each brings, Community-Based Participatory Research widens the angle of regard for public health activities, acknowledging community networks and leaders, Local knowledge of adverse social and economic consequences of environmental degradation and community beliefs and attitudes are all vital factors that directly impact the efficacy of research and community outreach. CBPR carries with a necessary mandate to restructure the undemocratic expert-client relationship because hypothesis, analysis and interpretation directly affects the social power dynamic".

Research concepts such as the Community-Based Participatory Research provide for a broader approach to the appreciation and integration of social learning systems as well as the structural inclusion of communal practices in achieving set goals. A social learning system thus, is typified by the expression of shared experiences in order to gain higher knowledge about a social phenomenon and the mobilization of concerted effort while observing historical, cultural and social factors that can increase competence and aid the learning process. Wenger, E. avers that "In a Social Learning System, competence is historically and socially defined. How to be a physicist or how to understand the position of the earth in the universe is something that scientific communities have established over time. Knowing therefore is a matter of displaying competencies defined in social communities. The picture is more complex and dynamic than that however. Our experiences of life and social standards of competence of our communities, are not necessarily, or even usually congruent. We each experience knowing in our own ways. Socially defined competence is always in interplay with our experience. It is in this interplay that learning takes place".

The Role of the community to learning and indeed transformation appear crucial to the overall notion of development in that they provide the enabling structures that should engender social activities needed for the transformative process to thrive. Scholars like Lave, Wenger and more recently Haneda have proposed that a community of practice perspective is instructive in underscoring the relationship between the individual and his immediate society. As a factor in situated learning, a community of practice mechanism ensures that knowledge and learning is socially acquired through the participatory process embedded in social-cultural activities. Mari Haneda observes that "For Lave and Wenger, knowledge is not something that is incrementally stored in an individual's mind; it is to be understood relationally, that is to say, as located in the evolving relationships between people and the settings in simply receive, internalize and construct knowledge in their minds but enact it as persons-in-the world participating in the practices of a socio cultural community. Accordingly, learning is an intrinsic and inseparable aspect of any social practice, not the goal to be achieved and it occurs when people engage in joint activity in CoP, with or without teaching".

Social interaction between members of a community generates the needed traction for intervening measures to be taken. These measures are expressed through activities and practices and can occur in stages. Etienne Wenger projects that the social learning systems as practiced in various communities could exercised in various form and levels such that individuals within the community observe modes of belonging that regulate as well as propel levels of participation in the creative and/or development process. The table enunciates these stages.

S/N		
1.	Engagement	Doing things together, talking, and producing artifacts (e.g helping a colleague with a problem or participating in a meeting). The ways in which we engage with each other and with the world profoundly shape our experience of who we are. We learn what we can do and how the world responds to our actions.

2.	Imagination	Constructing an image of ourselves, of our communities, and of the world, in order to orient ourselves, to reflect on our situation, and to explore possibilities (e.g. drawing maps, telling a story, or building a set of possible scenarios to understand one's options). Imagination here is used in sense proposed by Benedict Anderson (1988) to describe nations as communities: it does not connote fantasy as opposed to factuality. Thinking of ourselves as a member of a community such as a nation requires an act of imagination because we cannot engage with our entire essential to our sense of self and our interpretation of our participation in the social world.
3.	Alignment	Making sure that local activities are sufficiently aligned with other processes so that they can be effective beyond our own engagement. The concept of alignment does not connote a one-way process of submitting to external authority, but a mutual process of co-ordinating perspectives, interpretations and actions so they realize higher goals. (Wenger:227-228)

Thus, the utilization of social learning systems as embedded within communal practices are critical and are employed in the engagement of RehabDramatics within the applied theatre projects carried out and documented from the next chapter. This, along with the systematic introduction of theatrical activities were expected to increase individual as well as community participation in proffering solutions to the myriad of issues affecting special or 'closed' populations as seen in the cases of 'at risk' children and adolescents.

CHAPTER FOUR

DATA SOURCING AND PRELIMINARY RESEARCH ACTIVITIES FOR APPLIED THEATRE ENGAGEMENTS WITH REHABDRAMATICS

Four Applied Theatre workshops were carried out in selected institutions across two states in Nigeria, namely Edo and Anambra. In order to ensure a detailed system of data presentation as well as a holistic and empirical approach to the research work, the researcher engaged preliminary research instruments and activities which provided background information about the objective of the research work as well as the course of action in actualizing the individual-group projects. These activities are outlined as follows:

Consent forms/Approval letters: Since studies and engagements such as this would involve extensive interaction with participants who are in most cases children with special needs as well as their administrators, teachers, parents and care givers, it is expedient to obtain proper approvals for access within the scope of time for the research work. The approval letters, thus were designed to ensure that the consent of these somewhat closed populations were adequately sought and obtained. The letters include the contact details of the researcher and department, a brief summary of the research objective, the concepts, theories and methodology being relied upon, a brief outline of the process to be engaged and an attestation to protect the identities and privacy of the participants during the course of the project. (See Appendix 2).

Interviews: The researcher conducted a number of interviews in the course of the study. These interviews were either structured or unstructured depending on the approach utilized or the given circumstances available at the time of research. During the preliminary visits for instance, interviews were conducted with key officials of various institutions both related to and where the Applied Theatre projects were to be carried out. The sessions provided the researcher ample opportunity to explain in detail the objective of the research. Explanations on the rehabilitative potentials of dramatic activities were shared and espoused on. The inclusion of African Oral tradition such as indigenous folklore, games and songs were also explained as agents with instructive material through dramatic enactments; and as co-facilitators of rehabilitative and developmental change in *at-risk* individuals. In other instances, the interviews were also tailored based on the special composition and needs of the school or center being evaluated as at the period of research.

Plate 1

1A

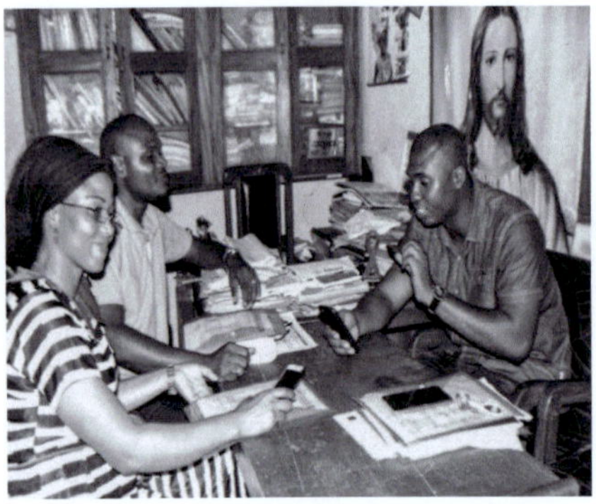

1B

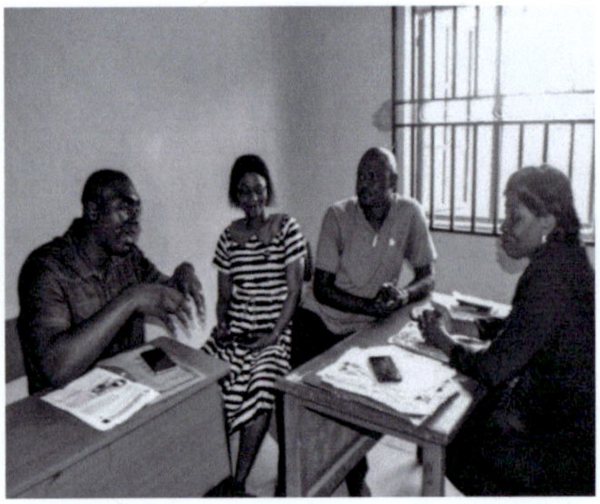

Interview sessions with officials from the ministry of Education and the Head teacher of the school of the blind Edo State

1C

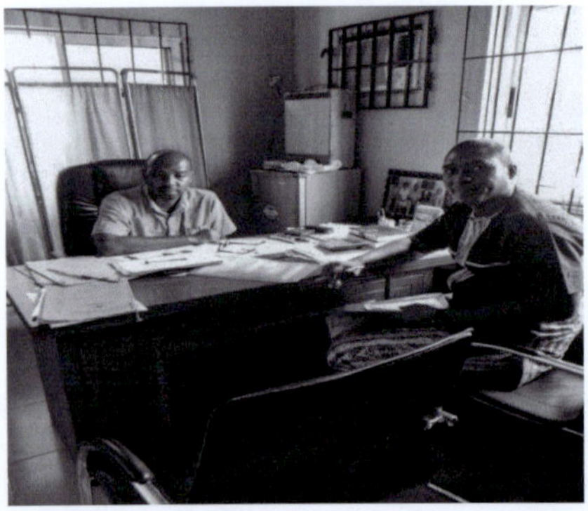

1D

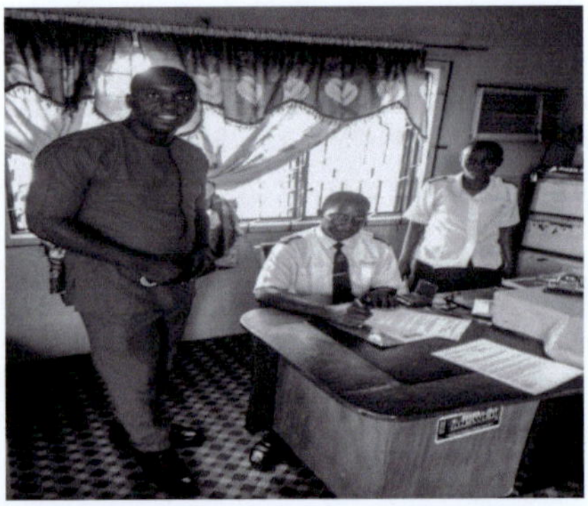

Interview sessions with the medical director of the psychiatric hospital Dr. C. C. Onuorah and with the director of the rehab centre Edo State Major Bramwell Chukwunwem

Advocacy Sessions: The Researcher also organized larger sessions with teachers, care givers and parents in the various locations where the projects were to take place. These sessions afforded the researcher the opportunity to explain the objective of the projects as well as to interact with the participants on the various socio-economic and environmental factors prevalent within the communities as they affect at risk children and adolescents. The sessions also include an appraisal of the Oral folk tradition in the communities and its importance to social *conscientization* and development. The essence of dramatic enactments as key tools in mobilizing needed support against certain phenomena, were also discussed. Mock rehearsals of indigenous folk games and songs were carried out to give the teachers and caregivers a contextual appreciation of the scope of the workshops. The researcher took down notes and learnt some of these indigenous songs and games. Oral consent was then sought to kick start interactions and rehearsals with would-be participants.

2A

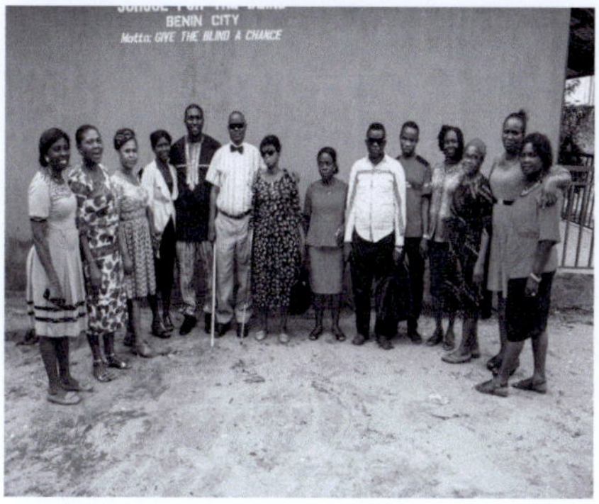

2B

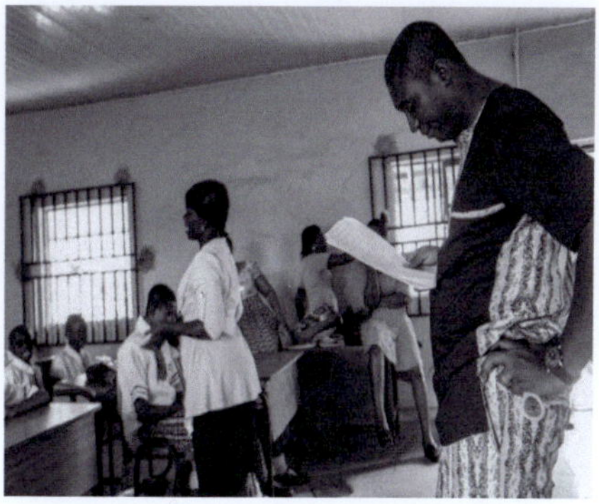

Advocacy sessions with some teachers and parents and initial interaction with the Participants

Preliminary Interactions with the Project Participants: Across the four locations where the Applied Theatre workshops are to be carried out, the researcher interacted with the participants and these sessions were either held in group settings or on one on one basis. Questions were asked on the acknowledgment, perceptions and tendencies towards certain phenomena such as stigma, bullying, societal norms and so on and how these affect the day to day living of at-risk children within the environment. The Researcher employed the Interpretative Phenomenological Analysis in inquiring from participants, particular experiences or perceptions of certain phenomena, how they affect them and the desired responses or behaviours they would properly want introduced.

Plate 3

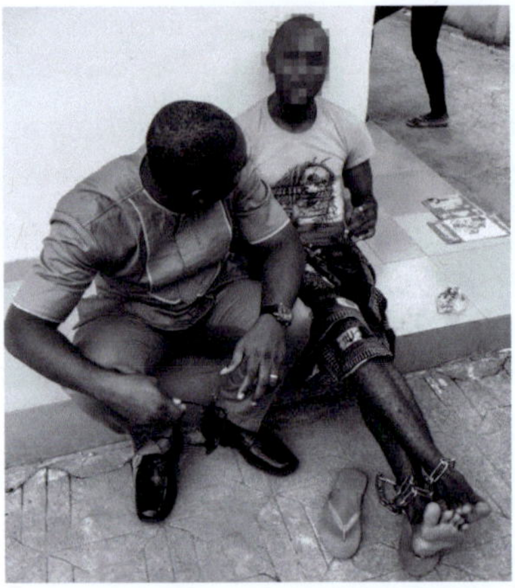

Interactive and story creation processes using IPA

Current Study Hypothesis: Based on the interactions carried out between the researcher, teachers, caregivers and the children-participants. The following hypotheses were formulated:

Hypothesis 1: Over the course of the workshop, participant dramatic engagement and involvement should increase.

Hypothesis 2: Therapeutic bonding that could foster rehabilitative change should occur.

Population of the Study: The Applied theatre projects were carried out across four locations in two states namely Anambra and Edo. The areas covered in Anambra include Amaenyi in Awka South Local Government area and Nawfia in Njikoka Local Government Area both within the Anambra central senatorial District of the state. The areas covered in Edo state are Oliha-Ivbiore and East Circular both in Oredo Local Government Area, Benin. The researchers, worked with a total of fifty two participants from the various locations covered. 20 students participated from God's Care Special School Amaenyi, 8 inmates participated from the Nawfia psychiatric Hospital, 10 pupils participated from the School of the Blind, Ivbiore and 14 inmates participated from the Salvation Army Rehabilitation Center.

Method of Data Collection: The researcher adopted the use of interviews and participant observation as major methods for data collection. These indepth interviews were presented in both structured and semistructured formats. The structured interviews allowed for a proper documentation of questions which the researcher adduced to be pertinent from interactions with the participants, to the mandate of the study. These questions were prepared beforehand and asked to individuals who could provide relevant insight to the research discourse. Participants of the various applied theatre projects were also asked particular questions in order to acquire first hand information on the personal perceptions on given phenomena. The semi structured interviews were occasioned by the need to attain better insight on new situations and understandings not earlier envisaged, as the research progressed. These were mostly oral and were particularly apt in eliciting individual experiences and sense-making of certain phenomena that were considered as factors within the various projects carried out as well as in the study in its entirety. The responses were mostly open ended, detailed and well supported suggesting considerable reflection and thought. The structured questions were administered after the productions to ascertain the occurrence of changes in perceptions and attitudes to given situations.

The research study engaged children and young adults who were pupils, students or inmates in the various establishments and communities surveyed, on a range of issues bothering on their perceptions towards contrived social constructs and behaviours as well as communal or cultural conjectures and attitudes towards individuals with similar disabilities. Questions on the acceptance to utilize dramatic and performance based activities in interrogating and questioning these belief systems as well as personal perceptions and attitudes to the various situations received mostly positive responses. The structured interviews were configured to cover the four research areas covered. In the areas where the participants were able to communicate with relative competence on issues concerning them independently, the researcher adopted a two pronged question-type format. However, even where the participants could communicate adequately but were unable to write down answers themselves because of their disability, the researcher and his assistants them; with further guidance of the care givers or teachers present. For three out of the four projects, a Type 'A' question format was used for the participants themselves, while Type 'B' was used for other concerned individuals such as Caregivers, Parents, Teachers, Doctors, Health care administrators, Policy makers and so on. Consequentially, Type 1A and B was adopted for the school of the Blind, Ivbiore, Edo State. Type 2A and B was adopted for the God's Care Special School, Umuayom – Amaenyi, Awka, Anambra State. Type 3A and B was adopted for the Psychiatric Hospital Nawfia, Anambra State while Type 4 was adopted for the Salvation Army Rehabilitative Center, Oredo, Edo State.

The questions administered also provided as a pre-test evaluation exercise. The researcher resolved to administer the same questions, especially those of significance to the research outcomes, after the productions in order to ascertain incidences of variance from pre- performance positions and beliefs. The researcher engaged this pre production and post production evaluation format particularly in the Ivbiore and Amaenyi projects; largely because both locations provided a more formal environment for predetermined and documentary outcomes to be attained. However, in the Nawfia and Oredo projects, evaluation question were mostly administered orally and documented by the researcher in the determination of research outcomes. Overall, changes in views, perception and reactions were calculated to indicate simple increase or decline in results. The presentation of the questions covered two major aspects namely an introductory section which included the demographic disposition of the respondents (see Appendix 1), and the answer section. Examples are given below;

INTERVIEW QUESTIONS
TYPE 1A (PARTICIPANTS)

S/No	
1	How old are you?
2	Where are you from?
3	Do you live with your parents?
4	Do you remember anything about how you lost your sight?
5	Are there specific challenges you go through as a result of your disability?
6a	What do you understand by the word, discrimination?
6b	Have you ever felt discriminated against because of your disability?
6c	How often does this occur?

6d	Have you been discriminated against by close friends and family members?
7a	What do you understand by the word, Bullying?
7b	Have you ever had to endure bullying because of your disability?
7c	How often does this occur?
7d	Have you ever been bullied by friends and family members?
8a	What do you understand by the word Molestation?
8b	Have you ever had to endure Molestation because of your disability?
8c	How often does this occur?
8d	Have you ever been molested by close friends and family members?
9	Do you like Acting, Dancing, Singing, Swimming etc?
10	Would you want to be part of a Theatre project?
11	Would you want us to act out your own story?
11b	How do you think people will react to it?
11c	Do you think your story can help someone with similar disabilities and challenges?
12	Do you know any folk song/game/dance?
13	Can you sing/play/perform any?
14	Do you understand the underlining meanings of these songs/games/dances?
15	Have you heard of any folk song/game/dances that says bad things about children who have lost their eye sight?
16	Have you learnt something new from this theatre project?
17	Do you want theatre projects like this to continue in your school?
18	Do you think children like you will like these type of performances?
18b	Do you think parents can learn from this kind of project?
18c	Do you think other members of society need to be part of this kind of project?

TYPE 1B

S/No	
1	Could you tell us who you are and what you do?
2	Are you a parent?
3	Do you have children who are visually impaired?
4	In your view, how has the society treated children with visual impairment? Examples?
5	Do you feel that our social attitudes and behaviour have put children with visual impairment at greater disadvantage?
6	Are children with visual impairment more likely to be bullied?
7	Are children with visual impairment more likely to be discriminated against?
8	Are children with visual impairment more likely to be molested or taken advantaged of?
9	Are the traditional customs and practices in your community supportive of issues of bullying, discrimination and molestation of children with visual impairment?
10	Are you open to the idea of using drama and theatre in x-raying these issues as they concern children with visual impairment?
11	Do you agree that secondary challenges which may be mental or psychosocial in nature, are more likely to occur in children living with visual impairment?

TYPE 2A (PARTICIPANTS)

S/No	
1	How old are you?
2	Were you born this way?
3	Do you live with both parents?
4	Do you have other siblings?

4b	Do you have siblings or close relatives with similar diability?
5	Do you believe that your disability is as a result of a spiritual attack?
6	Do people (your family inclusive) treat you differently because of your disability?
7	What do you understand by bullying and discrimination?
8	Have you ever been bullied because of your disability?
9	Have you been bullied by your peers with similar disabilities?
10	Do you bully your peers with similar disabilities?
11	Would you want to take part in a drama project on challenges faced by children with hearing and speech disabilities?
12	Would you be willing to share your story within the course of the project?

TYPE 2B

S/No	
1	Tell us about yourself?
2	Do you have children, relatives who have speech and hearing challenges?
3	What are your general perceptions about children with hearing and speech challenges?
4	Do you agree that biological and genetic factors could contribute to hearing and speech loss in children?
5	Do you agree that accident, mishap and some man-made factors can contribute to hearing and speech loss in children?
6	Do you believe that spiritual forces could be responsible for hearing and speech loss in children?
7	Do you agree that actions of discrimination against children with hearing and speech disabilities take root from communal practices, individual behaviour or both?

8	Are you aware of any special school, center, or facility that provides care for children with hearing and speech disability?
9	Would you recommend special education for children with hearing and speech disability?
10	Do you think that children with hearing and speech disability are more likely to be Bullied and discriminated against?
11	Do you think that children with these disabilities are more likely to get into vices such as stealing, violence etc
12	Are you aware of communal practices or social constructs that negatively affect children with these disabilities?
13	Do you know any child with these disabilities that has anger issues?
14	Do you think that dramatic activities can be used to engage children with hearing speech disabilities?
15	Would you recommend dramatic engagements with any child you know who has these disability?

TYPE 3A

S/No	
1	Tell us about yourself?
2	Why are you here?
3	How do you see yourself?
4	Do you like taking hard drugs?
5	Can you remember when you started taking it?
6	Why do you think your family brought you here?
7	Do people treat you differently?
8	How do people treat you?
9	How do you feel towards people that treat you badly?
10	Do you like watching Drama/Plays

11	Would you want to be part of a play?
12	Would you want us to act out your story through drama?

TYPE 3B

S/No	
1	Tell us about yourself
2	Do you know anyone who is mentally challenged?
3	What in your opinion are the causes of mental challenged in young Adult?
4	Do you believe that many of the cases in the psychiatric Hospital Nawfia were spiritually orchestrated
5	How many mental or psychological disorders are you aware of?
6	Do you think members of this community are aware of the various mental disorders that could effect individuals

The researchers in the course of the Amaenyi project, administered questionnaires in order to ascertain and determine quantifiable responses to the various perceptions and attitudes surrounding the understanding, acceptance and care of children with speech and hearing disabilities. The school used for the Applied theatre project is situated within the Awka metropolis, thus, the advantage of involving literate members of the community that would be able to understand thoroughly the subject of the research and communicate on same with some level of proficiency, provided cause to engage this instrument.

Subsequently one hundred and twenty adult respondents mainly comprising of parents, civil servants, professionals, traders, students and artisans were served questionnaires: thirty respondents were polled from the Amaenyi axis were the school is located, thirty were polled from the Aroma/ Okpuno axis, thirty were polled from the Ifite axis while another thirty were polled from the Nnamdi Azikiwe University community axis with the following statistics:

SECTION A (Demographic disposition of respondents)

Table 1: Age Range of the Respondents

S/N	AGE	NUMBER OF RESPONDENTS	PERCENTAGE OF RESPONDENTS
1	18 – 25	29	24.16%
2	26 – 39	54	45%
3	40 - Above	37	30.83%
	TOTAL	120	100%

Table 1, shows that 29 persons representing 26.16% of the respondents are between the ages of 18 – 25. 54 persons representing 45% of the respondents are between the ages of 26 – 39, while 37 persons representing 30.83% of the respondents are between 40 years of age and above.

Table 2: Distribution of Respondents according to gender

S/N	GENDER	Frequency	PERCENTAGE
1	MALE	57	47.5%
2	FEMALE	63	52.5%
	TOTAL	120	100%

Table 2, shows that 57 persons representing 47.5% of the total population surveyed are male, while 63 persons representing 52.5% of the population are female.

Table 3: Distribution of Respondents according to marital status

S/N	RESPONSE	NUMBER OF RESPONDENTS	PERCENTAGE OF RESPONDENTS
1	MARRIED	69	57.5%
2	SINGLE	51	42.5%
	TOTAL	120	100%

Table 3, shows that 69 persons representing 57.5% of the respondents are married while 51 persons representing 42.5% of the respondents are single.

Table 4: Educational Qualification of Respondents

S/N	QUALIFICATION	NUMBER OF RESPONDENTS	PERCENTAGE OF RESPONDENTS
1	WAEC	32	26.6%
2	BA/BSC/HND	63	52.5%
3	MA/MSC	17	14.16%
4	PhD	8	6.6%
	TOTAL	120	100%

Table 4, indicates the academic qualifications of the respondents as follows; 32 persons representing 26.6% possess senior school leaving certificates, 63 persons representing 52.5% possess BA/BSC or its equivalent. 17 persons representing 14.16% of the respondents possess an MA or MSC Degree while 8 persons representing 6.6% of the respondents are PhD degree holders.

Table 5: Distribution of the Respondents according to Occupation

S/N	OCCUPATION	NUMBER OF RESPONDENTS	PERCENTAGE OF RESPONDENTS
1	STUDENTS (MA & PhD)	25	20.83%
2	CIVIL SERVANTS/ PROFESSIONALS	54	45%
3	TRADERS/ ARTISANS	41	34.16%
	TOTAL	120	100%

Table 5, indicates that 25 persons representing 20.83% of the respondents are post graduate degree students. 54 persons representing 45% of the respondents are civil servants and professionals of different cadres, while 41 persons representing 34.16% of the respondents are traders and artisans.

The "My Mother's words" Project, School for the Blind. Ivbiore, Benin, Edo State

The Ivbiore project lasted for a cumulative period of 12 weeks at the School for the Blind, Ivbiore Benin, Edo State with a contact period of 2 sessions per week for 90 minutes each day. Ten primary 4 and 5 pupils were selected for the Applied Theatre project which comprised of 6 girls and 4 boys. Preliminary interactions which comprised of games, singing sessions, tales of personal experience and dramatic enactments, enabled the researcher with the assistance of teachers to select the children who exhibited greater willingness to be part of the project. The research team was charged to come up with story materials drafted from the experiences of the participants, while tailored to address themes such as stigma, rejection, abuse, forgiveness and Respect. There was a systemic infusion of performances as well as oral African traditional activities such as folk games, folklore, and folk songs and these were to be included as mid-scene additions as well as scene-changing mechanisms by the orchestra in order to further drive the messages behind the dramatic enactments. These folk songs, chants and poetic renditions provided not only needed embellishments in the play-making process, but also provided engaging activities for all the participants as the utilization of singing sessions and the likes, enhanced the effectiveness of sound and imaginative activities and thus allowed for a more participatory exercise.

General observations within the preliminary interactive and one on one sessions as well as interviews with the Head Mistress and teachers revealed that a greater number of the pupils of school were victims of congenital anomalies which were also offshoots of other issues related to birth defects and so on. Some of the pupils are diagnosed with anophthalmos or microphthalmos in which cases, the entire eyeball is smaller than normal or entirely absent from birth. The profiling drawn from the participants after 2 sessions for instance, reveals the following:

Participant	Pseudonym	Class/Age	Gender	Notes
Pupil 1	'Cherish'	5/12	Female	Congenital anomaly partial eyeballs visible
Pupil 2	'Sarah'	5/13	Female	Congenital anomaly
Pupil 3	Obi	5/12	Male	Congenital anomaly

Pupil 4	‘Chinenye	4/15	Female	Congenital anomaly Abandoned at a public Toilet at birth
Pupil 5	‘Malcom’	5/13	Male	Congenital anomaly
Pupil 6	‘Mary’	4/12	Female	Birth defect
Pupil 7	‘Nnenna’	5/13	Female	Premature birth
Pupil 8	‘Levi’	4/13	Male	Congenital anomaly
Pupil 9	‘Winner’	5/13	Male	Congenital anomaly
Pupil 10	‘Precious’	4/13	Female	Premature birth

Plate 4

4A

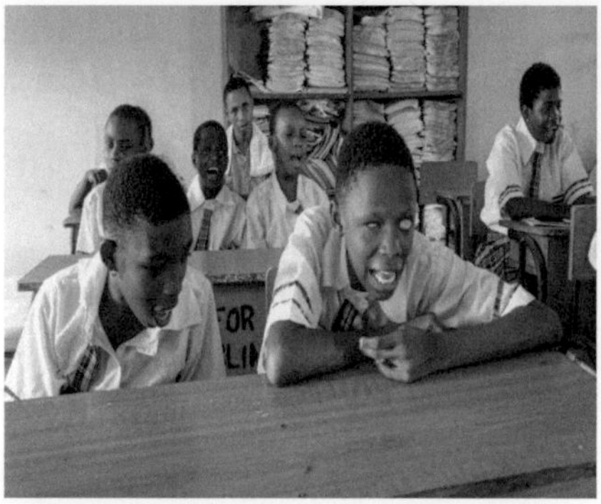

4B

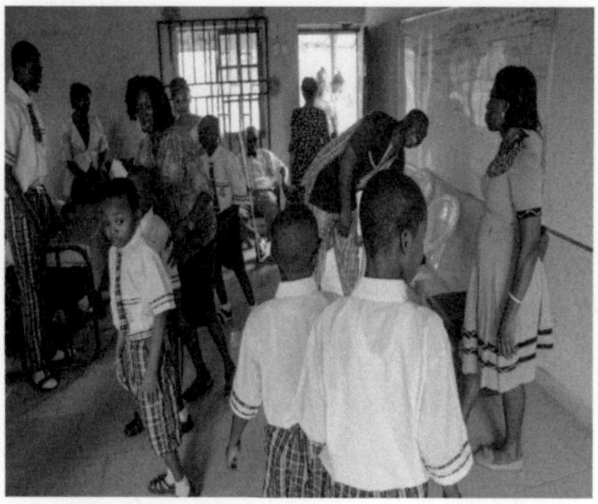

Cross Session of Pupils of the School of the Blind during Rehearsals

The participants of the project with the guidance of the researcher and teachers were able to create a story that was subsequently rehearsed through dramatic enactments. The story was developed drawing from the various interactive sessions with the participants and their teachers about individual experiences and perceptions on given phenomena. General observations were also taken into consideration about the societal and cultural conjectures and attitude towards various themes as it affects the average child in Edo state living with visual impairment. These issues range from, unplanned parenthood, societal discrimination, the concept of spirit children, poor educational facilities for children with special needs and so on.

The participants, thus, were able to create a five-scene play that was rehearsed over time. In scene 1 a middle aged woman is introduced: it is early morning. She is holding a lantern. She hears the cry of a newborn baby. She raises alarm and rallies neighbours within the vicinity and soon enough, a baby is discovered in a pit toilet nearby. The men of the community dig up the child. Everyone present express shock at sight of the baby. Unfortunately, maggots had eaten away at the baby's eyes. The young mother is identified. Mothers berate her. A song is raised on the pricelessness of children.

The second scene opens on a family meeting. The future of the young mother is being decided. The infant's Great grandmother offers to take care of the child so as to allow the young mother continue with her education. It is also revealed that the baby has lost her sight for good. In scene 3 teacher visits the home. She informs the grandmother of the child's exploits and canvasses for more support for the special child.

Scene 4 reveals the child coming home dejected. She expresses dismay on episodes of neglect and discrimination she encounters daily. She pledges hatred for so called 'normal' people including her mother for contributing to her state. Her Grandmother consoles her; she advises her and teaches her on the virtues of Love, understanding and forgiveness. She educates her on the travails of a mother and encourages her to be determined to make it in life (She sings, the orchestra joins in). In the last scene (*Years Later*), the girl is now a woman. She is accomplished and has just been appointed commissioner in her state. She gives a speech on the importance of diligence. She encourages other challenged youths present and calls up her mother to share the stage with her in a move for reconciliation and forgiveness (Her Great Grandmother has passed on). The scene ends with singing and dancing.

The "Free" Project, Psychiatric Hospital Nawfia

The project was initially drafted to span a period of maximum of 4 months due to the sensitivity of the research area. However, continued interaction appeared critical in gauging levels of social as well as dramatic engagements from the participants as the study progressed. There was a need to ascertain how changes observed could be sustained using dramatic activities as utilized within the research timeline. The project therefore lasted for a period six months with a 2-session weekly contact period lasting for about 1 hour each session.

8 participants aged between 15 to 26 indicated interest in joining the workshop after it was clearly explained to them with their parents or guardians present and with the assistance of the medical officers within the Hospital and research assistants. The sessions metamorphosed from interview stages with IPA[sic] to group discussions on given phenomena and then to theatrical engagements and activities which included games, songs, dances, role playing etc; which culminated into full blown rehearsals with a "statement" production in mind.

Observations emanating from preliminary interactive sessions and group discussions revealed a range of incidents and circumstances contributory to the plight of the participants. These factors ranged from effects of illicit drug and substance abuse to episodes of psychological breakdown resulting from a traumatic event such as the loss of a loved one and so on.

The group was profiled from the youngest as follows:

No	Pseudonym	Age	Gender	Notes
1.	"Glory"	15	Female	Was brought by a relative. accused of being a witch.
2.	"Blessing"	17	Female	Slipped into depression after giving birth.
3.	"Champion"	19	Male	Depressed after the loss of his father. Got involved in hard drugs.
4.	"Rich"	20	Male	Involved in Hard Drugs.
5.	"Peace"	21	Female	Receives regular treatment at the Hospital. Claims spiritual manipulation from extended family.
6.	"Dave'	23	Male	Suffers from bouts of depression. Claims to have been abandoned by family.
7.	"God's gift"	24	Female	
8.	"Bluesky"	25	Male	Claims spiritual manipulation by uncles. Lost his father & inheritance. Suffers from depression. Has written two novels.

Dramatic activities were introduced as the study progressed and this was geared towards increasing social awareness and participation. The researchers included activities such as folk games, dances, as well as singing and poem rendition sessions. By the fourth week the researcher along with his research assistants had begun the story creation process ahead of the theatrical production slated for April 2019.

Plate 5

5A

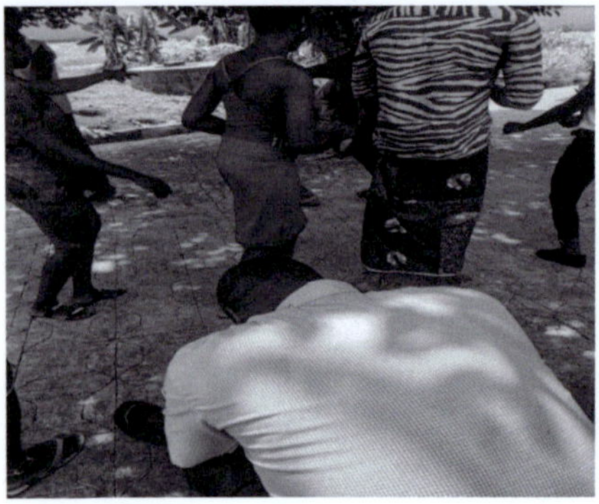

5B

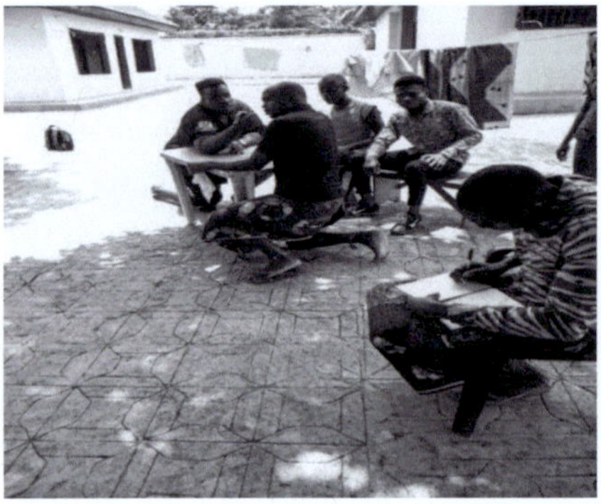

Rehearsal Engagements with the Participants

The production, a one Act Play centers on the various perceptions about inmates of the psychiatric hospital. The story x-rays the notion of depression as an outcome of other circumstances and choices within and outside the control of everyday people, as well as the need to see and explore good attributes amongst the inmates themselves through constructive and collaborative-group activities. The story revolves around Chuks also known as "Bluesky" who loses both parents tragically. The pain becomes too much for him and after episodes of nervous breakdowns, relatives "abandon" him at the psychiatric hospital. Within the hospital, he finds it difficult to associate with others and a couple of incidents make him even more withdrawn. Another character played as Kingsley helps Chuks to gradually increase his confidence in himself and in others; this is intermittently supported by songs and chants from the orchestra in driving home messages addressed within the play. The story hits a climax when Chuks, having found renewed vigour, defeats a bully aptly named "depression" in the Hospital in a mock – Arm wrestling contest but shows magnamity in victory by advocating for inclusiveness and cohesion in their common struggle against vices such as depression. There is a call by the narrator at the end of the play for communal effort in engendering more productive ways of accepting and working with persons who may have one mental challenge or the other. (see plate 15)

The "I am Special" Project, Amaenyi. God's Care Special School

The project was carried out at the school in Amaenyi, Umuayom; Awka South Local Government of Anambra State. The project involved working with the children in school, with the assistance of the school administration, teachers and research assistants in using the medium of drama to represent and assess different phenomena associated with the plight of challenged children especially as it concerns those with hearing and speaking difficulties. Initial observations revealed that while the major population of the children in the school suffered from different degrees of deafness and/or dumbness, the school has over the years, had to provide care for children with other challenges such as mental, biological and neurological deficiencies like Down syndrome, Albinism and so on. The project lasted for 3 months with a contact period of one hour daily, twice a week. Some of the students were noted to reside within the school premises for a number of reasons ranging from incidences of child abandonment to the total lack of specialized and constructive care for the said challenged children by their parents or guardians.

The purpose of the project was explained in detail at a special PTA session on the 20th of April, 2019 at which all the parents and teachers present were informed of the objective of the project. 18 students were selected based on their levels of willingness in engaging dramatic, playmaking and other theatrical techniques in aiding learning processes as well as evaluating issues concerning them. The students are profiled thus:

No	Pseudonym	Age	Gender	Notes
1.	"Samson"	11	Male	Deaf and Dumb. Has a twin brother who can hear and talk. Became deaf and dumb at age 7.
2.	Martha	12	Female	Deaf and dumb from birth
3.	"MJ"	12	Female	Deaf, dumb and mentally challenged slow in comprehension.
4.	J-Boy"	12	Male	Became deaf and dumb at the age of nine. Parents claim it is a spiritual attack. Dreams to be professional dancer or footballer.

5.	"Clara"	12	Female	Deaf and dumb abandoned as the school for 4 years.
6.	"Tim"	13	Male	Became deaf and dumb at age 4. Suffers from frequent bouts of convulsion.
7.	"Oprah"	13	Female	Deaf and dumb from birth.
8.	"Dave"	14	Male	Became deaf and dumb at 6. Family claims it is a spiritual problem.
9.	"Clems"	14	Male	Deaf and dumb from birth. Wants to be an engineer.
10.	"Joe"	14	Male	Mentally challenged. Suffers from down syndrome. Resides in the school.
11.	"Sammy"	14	Male	Deaf and dumb from birth. Wants to be a professional footballer.
12.	"Nuella"	14	Female	Deaf and dumb from birth. Was reported to have been affected by drugs the mother ingested during pregnancy
13.	"Mark"	14	Male	Deaf and dumb from birth.
14.	"Divine"	14	Male	Deaf, dumb and mentally challenged from birth.
15.	"Miracle"	15	Female	Deaf and dumb from birth.
16.	"Terry"	15	Male	Suffers from down syndrome.
17.	"Naomi"	16	Female	Deaf and dumb from the age of 7.
18.	"Bobby"	16	Male	Deaf and Dumb from the age of 9.
19.	"Vincent"	16	Male	Deaf and dumb from birth.
20.	Charity	17	Female	Deaf and dumb, became pregnant at 15. Abandoned by family. Resides in the school after her baby was adopted.

The research group adopted a story creation process that would engage the participants individually and as a part of the group. The overall performance took a quasi-pantomimic approach; this was in order to surmount the hurdle of communicating through speech which many of the participants were challenged with. However, some of the other activities such as singing & dancing within the project were carried uninterrupted and intermittently while the wordings of the songs were both translated through sign language and inscribed on card board paper for the benefit of larger audience. Through initial interactive and interview sessions with the aid of IPA[sic], researchers were able to extract workable thematic materials for the Applied drama play project, these include challenges posed by Bullying, diverse socio cultural constructs and perceptions, inadequate knowledge on the learning needs of children with hearing and speech difficulties and so on. Dramatic representations of these themes were infused in the rehearsals and participatory engagements that followed.

Plate 6

6A

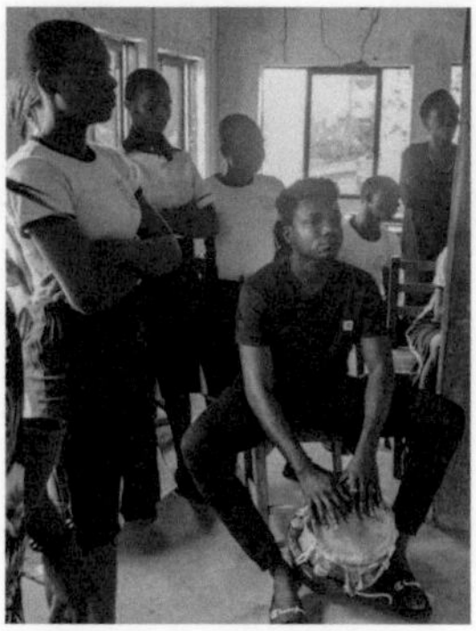

6B

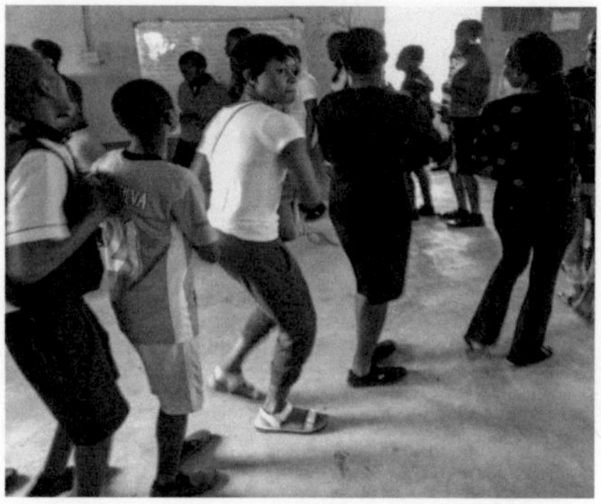

Rehearsals with Creative Activity Using Dance Movements and Mime

6C

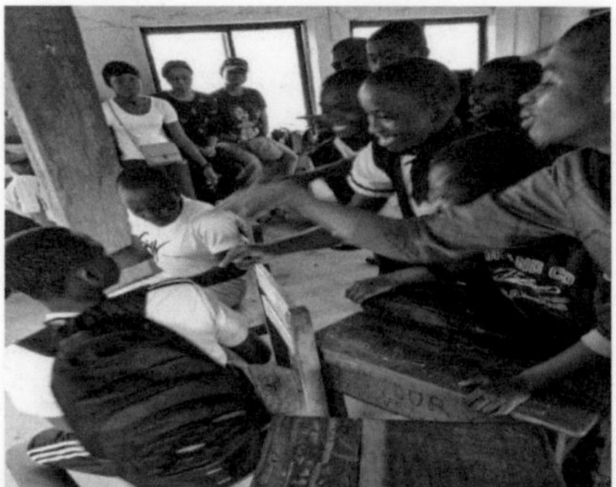

6D

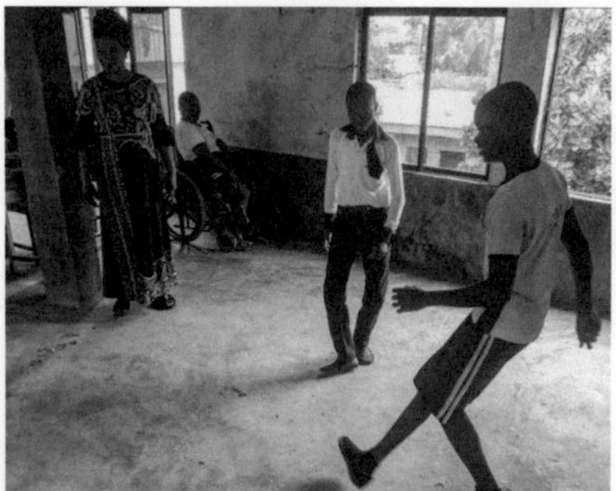

Scene Creation Processes with the Aid of Sign Language

6E

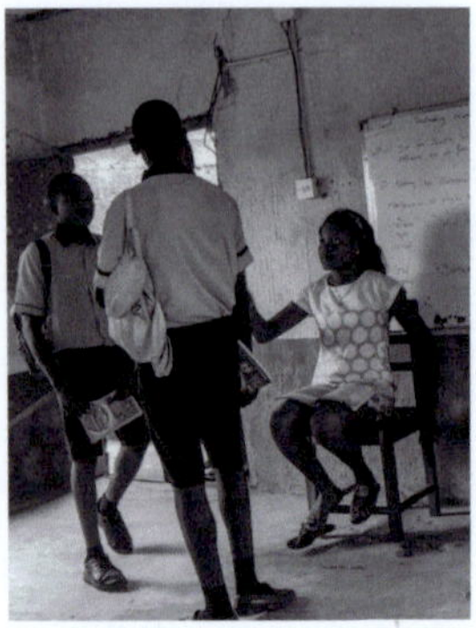

6F

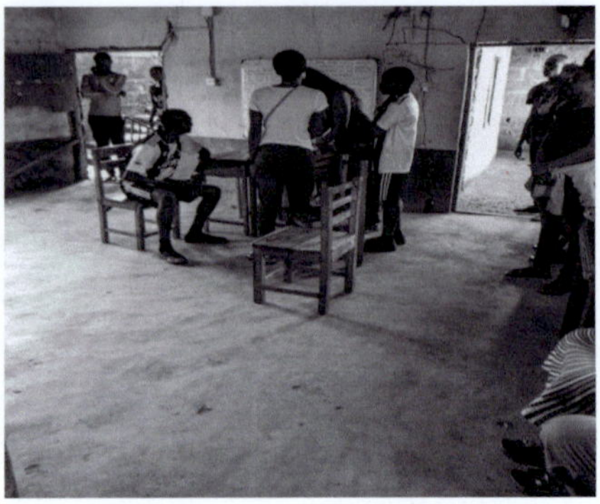

Rehearsing Dramatic Representations of the Menace of "Bullying"

The eventual story created tells of "J-boy" a boy who grapples with the menace of bullying and discrimination within and outside his school. This causes him to develop a low esteem of himself as evidenced in outbursts of anger and frustration. In the first scene, we are introduced to J-boy's predicament where he is refused from joining a game of football with his peers because of his disability. He engages in a fight before his brother wades in. in scene 2, the fight incident, which is one among many, is reported to J-boy's mother who is obviously exasperated about the plight of her son. The situation takes more challenging angles as the boy's father believes that his son's case is a spiritual one and that the gods may be out to cause his family harm through his son. To further make things worse, J-boy's grades continue to drop in the face of continued depression and frustration. In the penultimate scene, a friendly neighbour advices the family on the need for specialized care and training for J-boy. The family agrees and books an appointment with the school administration. Months later, there are remarkable changes in J-boy including renewed self belief and expression, improved cognitive abilities and better grades. The play comes to an end with a call to parents, guardians and children themselves to seek proper and inclusive ways to improve the well being of the challenged child.

The "Be Kind" Project, Salvation Army Rehabilitation Center, Oredo Edo State

The Salvation Army Rehabilitation center is located at Oredo, Edo State. Cited close to the Salvation Army Church as a mission project to the community, the facility houses children and Adolescents with various health challenges especially with regard to physical and mental disabilities. A greater percentage of these individuals who also reside at the center, are from Edo State while others come from different states in the country. The Applied Theatre workshop-initiative was explained to the Director and other officials of the center. The researcher also interacted with some would be participants to ascertain levels of willingness to be part of the project as well as to understand the peculiarity of challenges each individual is faced with. In further interactive sessions' that followed, participants zeroed in on addressing themes of bullying and discrimination hence, the workshop title, "Be kind". The project thus adopted the engagement of storytelling sessions embellished with performative dramatic actions repeated intermittently to engender retained interest. The workshop lasted 2 months with no final production in mind for a contact period of 90 minutes, once every week.

"Be kind" is a fictitious tale about an arrogant prince in a faraway kingdom who treats everyone around him with disdain and disrespect. He is very unlike his younger brother who is kind hearted, humble and respectful to elders. With the demise of their father, the king of the land, the community is thrown into worry and fear over the arrogant prince becoming king over them. However on the day of coronation, just as the crown prince is about to be crowned, the chief priest halts the ceremony and with the help of the people subdues and banishes the arrogant prince from the land. The kind and good natured prince is then crowned in his place and the people live happily ever after.

Plate 6

6A

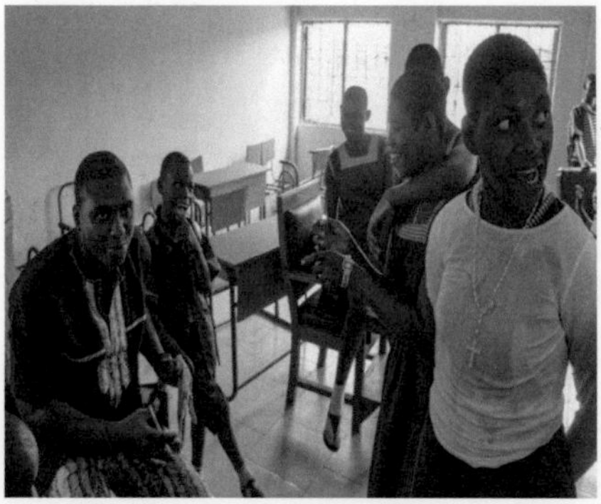

6B

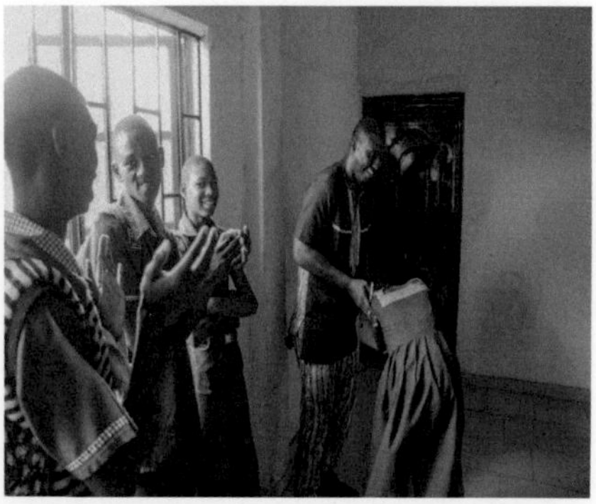

CHAPTER FIVE

REHABILITATIVE APPROACHES THROUGH DRAMA IN THE *IVBIORE*, *NAWFIA*, *OREDO* AND *AMAENYI* PROJECTS

The project attempted not just to raise the awareness of the socio-cultural factors as they affect the pupils, teachers and parents within and around the various communities studied, but also attempted to mobilize concerted effort by these stake holders and others in critically evaluating the effects of the issue arising alongside prospects for positive and holistic psycho-social development through the instrumentality of Drama.

One of the research instruments as earlier stated and utilized in the course of the project is the Interpretative Phenomenological Approach. This approach entails a detailed appraisal of the various phenomena *vis a vis* ideological and socio-cultural constructs that have affirmed themselves within the fabrics of the communities being researched and thus have shaped the conceptualization of certain notions and attitudes of the individuals within that community. In instances where these notions are linked to issues of health and physical wellbeing, IPA provides as an avenue to inquire and provide depth over a range of issues and experiences while putting them in context with present realities. Robert Allan et al agrees when he says that "IPA in particular can add mesh to the bones of a phenomenon, drill down and explore the depth of an issue for a particular group of people, further explore the nuances of the impact of context on relationships, or bring narratives to the fore, that explicate clinical challenges that cannot always be met with a singular treatment approach. Currently, there is also substantive dialogue about how research can contribute to improved clinical outcomes and evidence based practices".

The IPA approach, within the construct and application of Applied-Theatre processes and activities, thus provides an avenue for the participants to relive certain experiences with a view to contextualize the meaning and understandings ascribed to the phenomena responsible for them. Dramatic activities should therefore increase communal awareness about these phenomena and the attributed experiences; and where these activities are carefully guided to participants whose physical wellbeing are greatly affected by certain social attitudes, therapeutic change should occur. Dima reports on a Psychodrama study using IPA "Some examples drawn from IPA studies in different fields are: How does a woman's sense of identity change during the transition to motherhood? How do people who have complained about their medical treatment make sense of being angry? How do parents manage the challenges of living with an autistic child? What does jealousy feel like? The psychodrama study using IPA reported in this paper was guided by the following research questions; how do members of psychodrama therapy experience and make sense of therapeutic change? How do they experience and describe the group experience?".

The Ivbiore Project provided ample opportunities to relive certain experiences using dramatic activities and exercises. The researcher engaged participants in numerous one on one as well as group sessions. In some instances during the story-creation process, particular actions were dramatized either by the participants or the researcher to give the group a sense understanding of the reality and magnitude of each phenomenon as well as gauge the level of acceptance or otherwise of same.

These activities further engendered the utilization for relational group processes as an aspect of Drama therapy. This does not only seek the acknowledgement of certain phenomena and social attitudes prevalent in the society, but also gives attention to the specific needs of affected individuals who are victims of a system but yet are unique and distinct in levels of self-definition, expression, interest and so on. Richard Erskine opines that "Relational group psychotherapy often begins with recognizing each person's needs and feeling. The leader often encourages group members to focus on each person's need for security. That is the freedom to be as he or she is without criticism ridicule or put-downs. One of the first steps in healing stress, undoing cumulative neglect and resolving trauma is for each person to be assured that he or she will not be shamed in the group".

He further states that "Along with encouraging such confirmation, the group leader supports each in the group in expressing his or her uniqueness. People have the relational ability to know and express their own self-definition, individuality and distinctness while receiving acknowledgement and acceptance from others in the group. Self definition is the communication of one's self-chosen identity, the expression of preferences, interests and ideas without humiliation or rejection. In some family and school situations, children's attempts at self-definition are ridiculed or punished. When self definition is thwarted, internal stress increases and a sense of one's self is lost".

In the *Nawfia* and *Amaenyi* projects, the issues of stigma, discrimination and in some cases, exploitation were also examined. Some participants expressed how they have been misunderstood and discriminated against even by individuals they feel should know better. The "play" experience afforded them the opportunity to tell those present who they are and what they are not. In the dramatic piece at the Nawfia Psychiatric Hospital, "Uju" gives voice at defining herself "I am beautiful within and outside. I am special. I am not limited by my situation or hindered by my environment. I appreciate God who created this world and thought it wise to put me in it".

In the Amaenyi project, another participant makes a stand at self definition when he tells his audience through sign language "I refuse to let challenges stop me in life. I know within myself that I am not useless. I will study hard and achieve my dreams".

Plate 8

8A

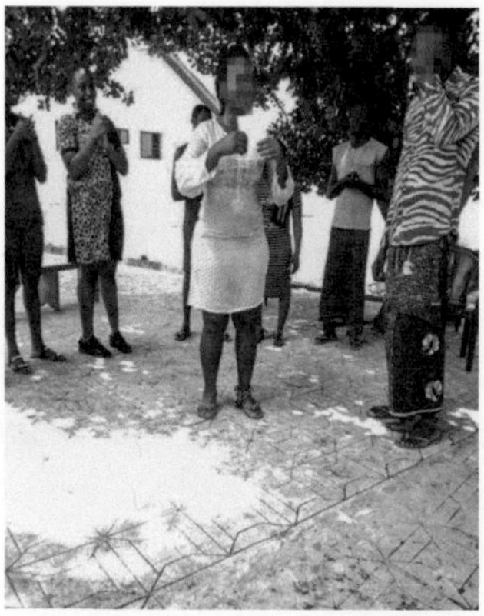

One of the *Nawfia* participants' attempt at self definition

8B

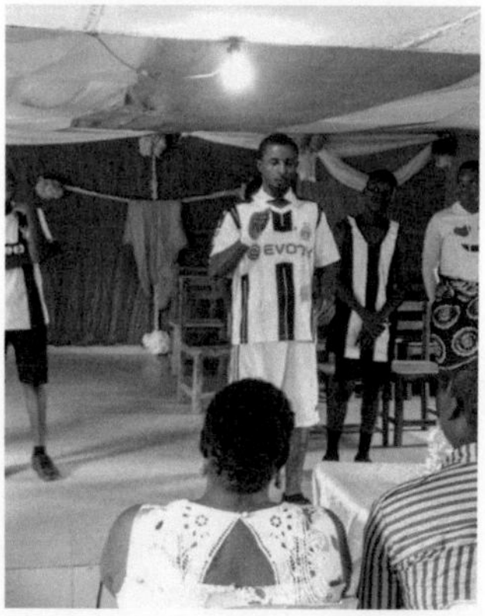

One of the *Amaenyi* participants attempt at self definition

The "Ivbiore" project developed the story along the experiences of the participants as well as the prevalent phenomena and social attitudes within the community and its environs. One of such issues is the spate of teenage pregnancies which scholars record to be on the increase in Nigeria. The phenomenon also appeared to be contributory to incidents of child mortality and other related challenges within the population studied and thus, formed a thematic component of the eventual workshop.

In the opening scene, we are introduced to one of the many effects of the mismanagement of Teenage pregnancy: a newly born baby is dumped in a public pit toilet and before the infant is rescued, some damage has been done which includes the loss of the baby's sight. To emphasize the enormity of the issue, the following line is rendered by one of the characters "children are priceless. They are gifts from God. Why didn't you give her to me my daughter? My back is not too weary to carry her."

Scholars uphold that certain phenomena indeed have given impact on society as well as on the response of its inhabitants to other individuals and situations. These factors are capable of influencing not just immediate reactions but also long term social behavior. David white observes that "One of the most important aspects of social phenomena is that it involves one person's observable behavior influencing another person. For example, racism is a social phenomenon because it is an ideology that people have constructed that directly affects another group forcing them to change their behaviours. There are many different ways that other people can influence or change our lives, but among them behavioural phenomena is probably one of the most significant".

Another of such factors emphasized in the group project is the phenomenon of stigma as it relates to the development of visually impaired children and adolescents. Observations reveal that quite a number of the participants of the project have had their fair share of incidents of stigma and discrimination as a result of the challenges they encounter being visually impaired. The instrumentality of dramatic activities, as an ensemble art form, thus, enabled the participants and facilitators to examine these challenges both on personal levels and as a group.

The creation and development of the story for the project afforded the participants the opportunity to express themselves on the different episodes of stigmatization and discrimination they have been made to endure within and outside the school environment. Some incidents that appeared to have shaped or induced certain responses from the participants and have been evaluated during the pre-production processes were re-enacted within the play. In one instance, one of the participants "Chinenye", recounts how a street neighbour always bellows at her whenever she goes to school using the phrase "The blind girl!" In other instances, people have used phrases such as "that blind girl that walks funny". These and many more appear to have made an impact on how she interacts with people especially those she meets for the first time. In the fourth scene with her 'grandmother', the following conversation ensues:

Chinenye: My inability to see them allows them say things about me. I do not know how the way I walk amuses them. They do not even know me.

Grandma: Don't let what people say define you. There is so much you have to offer. There is a reason you are here my child. You are an answer to us. And I am blessed to have you as my grandchild.

Chinenye: But sometimes mama, I wish I was never born. Why was I born only to be rejected? Why did my mother do it…

Grandma: Never blame your mother. The travails of motherhood are many. You are a Gift and nobody can deny us the blessing your life has brought us. There is a song our people sing, it reminds us of the wonders of children and the price our mother paid to carry us. Never blame your mother my child. (A song is raised).

Plate 9

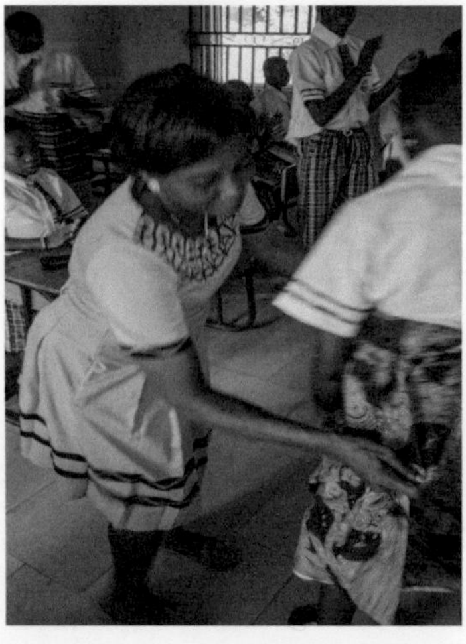

Integration of Folk Performance into the Dramatic process

The use of oral and performative activities, provide an atmosphere for messages intended to foster behavioural and psychosocial changes to thrive. Indeed within the African milieu, these cultural art forms have been observed to possess instructive materials in dealing with traumatic experiences as well as engendering increased social involvement. Addressing the confluence points between oral art forms and the dramatic medium as expressive channels of dealing with traumatic experiences with regard to the Rwanda Genocide, Chantal Kalisa defines oral cultures as "a natural tool for expressing the unspeakable nature of genocide and promoting recovery in post conflict societies" (n.pag). She further observes that "Theatre helps to recover voice and restore language. As such, drama acts as a Carthasis for survivors of genocidal violence by transforming their collective traumatic experience into art. With its healing potentials, theatre breaks the silence of trauma victims through body performances of physical reenactment/representations of violence. This embodied experience allows performers and the audience to envision new imagery and new language as well as to reconnect with "rituals" that were destroyed by genocide".

The integration of oral and performative art forms prevalent within the communities where the Applied Theatre projects held provides avenues for expressions of shared beliefs on certain phenomena. The intermittent use of folk songs and dances at intervals sought to drive home salient points discovered and evaluated during the pre-production processes. The integration of oral art forms such as the folk medium into the play making process formed an integral part of discussions and was deliberately infused as a mechanism to foster socio-cultural cohesion and interaction as well as an increase dramatic participation, self awareness and rehabilitation. In the Nawfia project, the researchers engaged folksongs and games within the rehearsal periods and utilized them as scene changing mechanisms in the eventual production. Examples of folksongs interlaced with dancing and dramatic activities include:

Onye bu Nwannem	Who is my sibling?
Ayoro Mma Mma Ayoro	Chorus
Emeka bu Nwannem	Emeka is my sibling
Ayoro Mma Mma Ayoro	Chorus
Mma no n' iru	He is handsome within
Ayoro Mma Mma Ayoro	Chorus
Mma no n' azu	He is handsome outwardly
Uju bu Nwannem	Uju is my sister
Ayoro Mma Mma Ayoro	Chorus
Mma no n' iru	She is beautiful within
Ayoro	Chorus

Mma no n' azu	She is beautiful outwardly
Ayoro mma mma	Chorus till fade
Ayoro ma yoro yo	
Ayoro mma mma Ayo	

These songs were accompanied with drumming and dancing activities to engender more inclusive involvement from the participants. However, some participants were observed to have increased participation as the rehearsal processes progressed. This could be classified into stages of indifference, partial participation and then to full participation and engagement.

Plate 10

10A

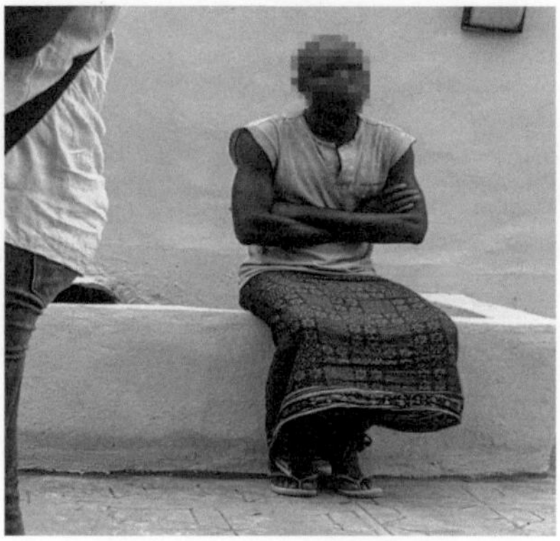

Initial state of indifference

10B

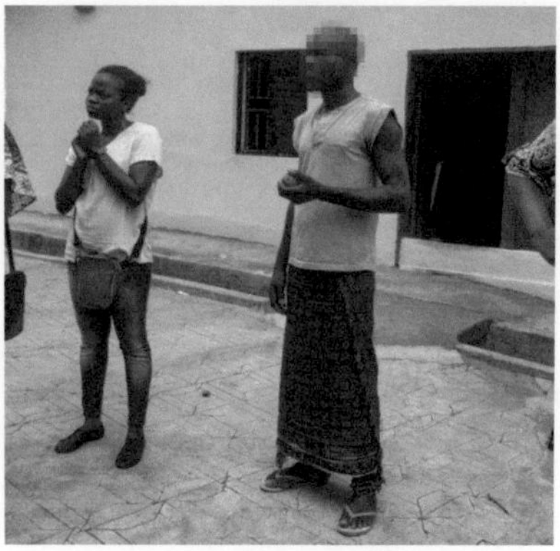

Partial involvement

10C

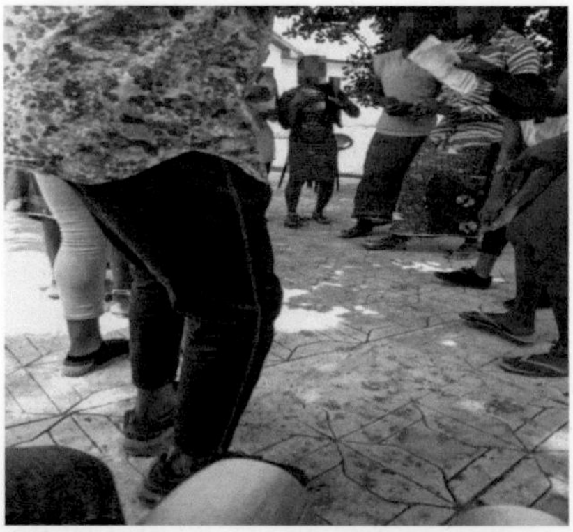

Fuller engagement and participation

Activities at the salvation army rehabilitation center, *Oredo* provided researchers and participants unique perspectives in adopting interactive techniques that would foster increased engagements and participation. Observations within the first 2 weeks revealed that though 14 children and young adults had indicated interest in participating in the Applied drama workshop, physical exertions, mobility and cognitive comprehension posed a significant challenge. For children with mental challenges such as Down syndrome and so on, the ability to remember actions or words learnt in previous sessions proved too much in some circumstances. However, having adopted performative storytelling sessions in which elaborate dramatic actions and gestures were intermittently infused, increased reactions and imitations were elicited. The researchers infused activities such as games, singing sessions, panthomime and dramatic representations in order to engender qualitative participation as well as evaluate individual response to certain themes, beliefs and practices. Indeed, these artistic activities were developed and carried from within the community; utilising their artforms in songs, chants, poetry and so on. The songs were taught with the assistance from members of staff and the participants themselves. One of the songs learnt in *Oredo* reads thus;

Waya Kugbe Oh

Song	Translation
Waya kugbe oh	Everyone let's come together in unity
Waya ko kugbe	It is God that created all of us
Waya kugbe	Both those that can see/walk
Osalobua oyi maya	And those that can't
Ke ne hia o	We are all one in the sight of God
O ke n nhia	
Osalobua eh moyi maya oh	

The use of indigenous folksongs in the performance creation process was also evident at the *Ivbiore* project. These songs mostly from *Bini* origin aided in driving home thematic and ideological messages on various concepts ranging from fate, motherhood, belief in God and others. Some of the *Bini* songs used in the production read thus:

Iye Mwen no Koko Mwen

Song	Translation
Iye Mwen nọ Koko Mwen	My mother that took care of me
Ke egbo omo bọ mwen gha de	From conception till now
Nọ ye iyeke vbo vbo mwen	The one that carried me on her back
Obe vba rhu ye mwen	Weldone mother!
Me tui iye mwen ọbe vba rhu	I salute you mother. Weldone!
Vbi idigue ke vbi uo vbie	I will kneel in honour of my mother
Ohan ghi gu mwen gui iye mwen	I will never talk back at my mother
Ghan emwen dan o	
Awuao awuao awua o	It is forbidden, it is forbidden, it is forbidden

Iye Okute

Song	Translation
Iye okuta edede mwen ede	Mother is a Rock
Nai se ti ghiyi I gho de	The one you cannot buy with money
Okhan vban mwen lu kui irhinhin	She carried me for nine months in her womb
Ovbo vbo mwen hu ukpe eha	And carried me on her back for three years
Iye okuta edede mwen ede	Mother is supreme.
Nai se tin ghi iye igho de	

Afiebe Vba

Song	**Translation**
Solo: A fien ebe vba ni o	Solo: who is cutting trees there?
Resp: kue kue	Resp: it is me
Solo: me no o	Solo: what are you doing with wood?
Resp: kue kue	Resp: it is me
Solo: vbu aye ebe rhu	Solo: what are you doing with wood:
Resp: kue kue	Resp: I want to build a house with them
Solo: Ti khan ya bo owa o	Solo: what do you want to do with a house?
Resp: kue kue	Resp: I want to marry and put a wife in it
Solo: vbo ayo owa rhu	Solo: what do you want a wife for?
Resp: kue kue	Resp: she would bear me wonderful children
Solo: Ti whe no bie men o	Solo: what do you want children for?
Resp: kue kue	Resp: children are a blessing to one.
Solo: vbu a ye omo rhu	
Resp: kue kue	
Solo: Omo rhu e mwin no omwan o	
Resp: kue kue	

The use of folk media within the dramatic process seeks to validate the communal perception of certain phenomena and thus foster a sense of consciousness on what is expected from society in dealing with these issues to forestall a possible breakdown of order or the loss of the virtue of humaneness within the society. Within performance, it is observed that folk songs possess distinct functionality in conveying deep messages as well as increasing dramatic action and participation within the developmental process. Ikenna Onwuegbuna observes that "although the functionality of music can be ascertained from a myriad of perspectives, it is in the textual content and performance practices of folk songs that the general world view of a people is exposed"(1). The essence of creativity within the application of folk media also provides as a veritable spectrum for transformation and rehabilitative endeavours to be engendered. Jakobson and Bogatyrev state that "Creativity is expressed here as much as in the selection of appropriated works as in their adaptation for other conventions and expectations. Established literary forms following their transference to folklore, become the raw materials for transformation".

The songs utilized in the "Ivbiore" project were raised by the Ochestra made up of Teachers, parents and pupils of the songs. These songs promoted a show of communal acceptance or rejection of given social phenomena. The interludes also allowed for participants to re-enforce their approval or disapproval of certain societal issues, attitudes and responses arising from the light of 'at risk' individuals. The projects also attempted to evaluate issues arising from established communal perceptions towards challenged children and adolescents. A common observation across the various projects revealed a very tangible belief system in the potency of spiritual manipulation of one sort or the other quite akin to the "spirit children" phenomenon in some areas in Southern Nigeria as well as in some parts of Africa. Indeed, while some community members believe that human actions could be contributory to issues of teenage pregnancy, child mortality, abuse and so on, there appears to be an adjoining belief in the frailty of the human nature against the whims of the supernatural and/or fate. For instance, quite a number of parents, and guardians in the various interactive sessions held expressed perplexity as to why a child would go deaf and dumb at the age of 9 or why out of four children born to seemingly healthy parents, one child would be stricken with degenerative health problems such as Down syndrome and so on. Applied Theatre workshops could be engaged in putting various ideologies in context while advocating for a course of action that would be beneficial to everyone. Mbachaga reminds us that "It is imperative to emphasize here that while we use Theatre to empower, we as practitioners should not ask people to change or do things that they don't want to do. This is because when Theatre "opens the eyes" of the people or target groups-conscientizes – the next thing is doing what they have learned – the action phase. However, doing or changing as a result of what they (individuals or communities) have discovered through the Theatre is a matter of choice".

The *Amaenyi* project laid these choices with a view to give perspectives to already held beliefs so as to foster a course of action in improving the quality of life of children with hearing and speech challenges.

Plate 11

11A

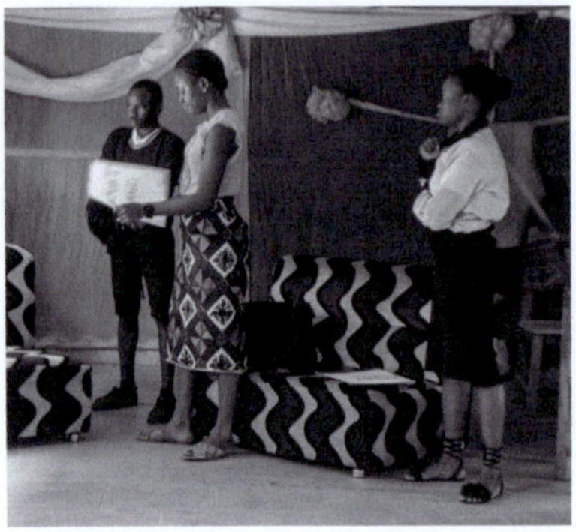

Mother is deeply unhappy about J-boy's grades and anger issues

11B

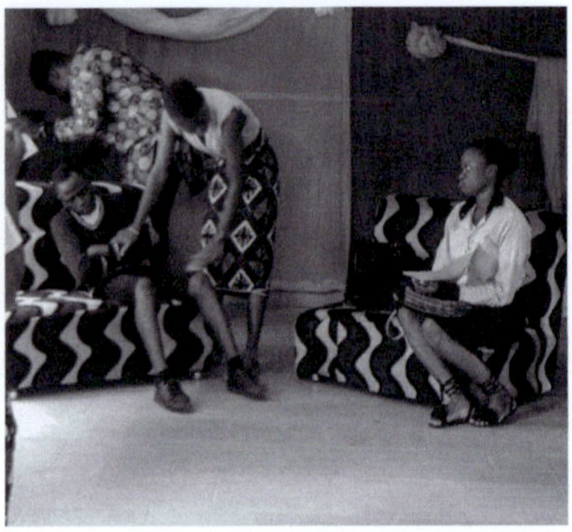

Father expresses concern on J-boy's predicament being spiritual

11C

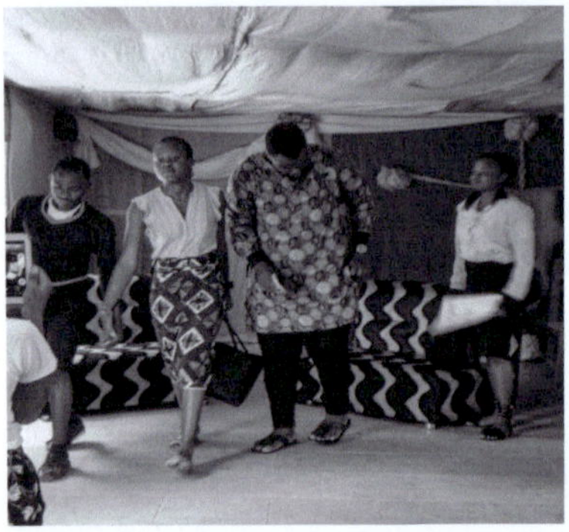

Decisive step to take concrete action

11D

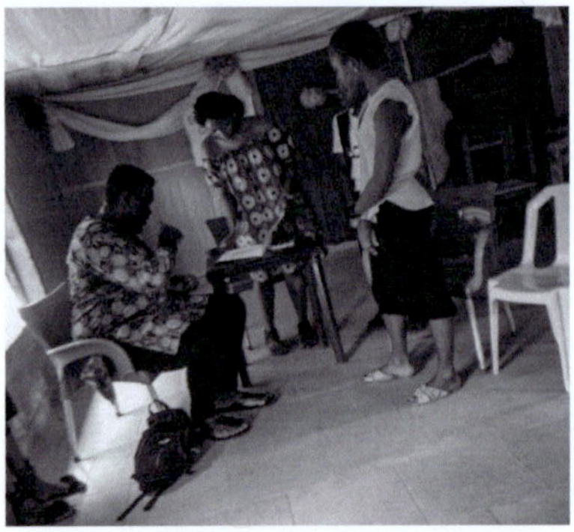

Father puts pen to paper to give specialized training for J-boy

The four Applied Theatre Projects utilized dramatic engagements and activities suited for each situation in assessing and evaluating general participation within processes of story creation and eventual performances. The projects also evaluate the impact of oral traditional art forms within the creative/rehabilitative process. Across the four research projects, observations revealed a seeming under-appreciation of the plight of challenged children and young adults and the need to engender proactive, qualitative and inclusive avenues to engage these individuals and non-disabled members of community. The approach of RehabDramatics thus, moves to be a medium for the engagement of arts in evaluating behaviour borne out of stereotypical, socio-cultural and communal conjectures such that peculiarities related to the varied forms of disabilities and challenges are better understood and represented. Rose Jacobson and Geoff McMurchy state that "Stereotypes surrounding disability have dominated the world of art, myth and historical imagery. Twentieth century depictions alone remind us of the tasks that lie ahead for those working to change attitude and representations" (3). Quoting Kazumi Tsuruoka, Jacobson and McMurchy Query further "What does integration mean in a society where the disabled are still largely seen as "freaks"? I have become a radical. I believe that nothing short of revelation can transform the collective mindset of my non-disabled brothers and sisters. Fear is the biggest obstacle to freedom and I am no longer afraid to be seen. I'm not asking you to like me, only see me as I am. Prepare for relationship, not symbols. That is what I have to offer".

The effectiveness of Applied drama in causing attitudinal, behavioral and psychological change in challenged children was constituted as one of the objectives of this study. The various projects infused thematic materials and activities that brought these issues to the front burner. In the *Ivbiore* and *Amaenyi* projects, though congenital problems and inherited biological anomalies could be traced as root causes of the disabilities of the participants, communal practices and beliefs were factored as capable of affecting and even complicating behavioural and psychological development in challenged children. Dramatic activities thus allowed for an evaluation of the practices and beliefs in context so as to create new perspectives to hitherto held positions. At the school of the Blind, *Ivbiore*, the Head teacher Mrs. Blessing Idede reports in an interview "Some of these children are actually susceptible to incidents of abuse and molestation. We have had a number of cases that are not very wonderful to the ears and yes, these have formed the way they behave. Many of them shy away from certain situations due to previous experiences. It is quite worrisome because our culture as a people does not support acts of molestation and discrimination".

During the post production discussions, another point was also raised on the need to properly define the disabilities children of the school suffer from. This point was discussed from the various interactions with some participants such as "Chinenye" who had been called "blind girl" on a number of occasions. It was generally agreed that the school name: "School of the Blind" *Ivbiore* did not conform to the move to reduce discriminatory references to the pupils as well as with regard to internationally accepted practices for special institutions of this nature. It was then agreed that a letter be sent to the commissioner of Education, Edo State for a change of name to "School of the Visually Impaired" whereas upon approval, a signboard bearing the new name should be erected by concerned community members. The approval has long been given and the sign board, erected. (See plate 12)

At the *Amaenyi* projects, the major issues revolved around incidences of spiritual manipulation and peer-bullying as factors affecting qualitative development in the children living with hearing and speech challenges. The rehearsal processes leading up to the eventual production afforded the participants avenues to give objective interpretations to these anomalies through expressive segments and representations. Some of these issues themselves also cropped up within the rehearsal sessions thus allowing for the researchers to address them immediately. One of the instances was the constant jeering at a female participant "Miracle" who exhibited extreme shyness and made some forceful grunting sounds whenever she stood up to 'say' something. This always elicited laughter from some other equally challenged members of group. The researchers were able to communicate the participants on the disadvantages of such responses, by deliberating infusing actions and gestures to discourage such behaviour while encouraging children like "Miracle" whenever they expressed themselves; there was an introduction of a reward system mechanism to engage these children in social and performative activities like dancing, games etc. geared towards improving confidence levels. (See plate 2).

In the *Nawfia* project, progressive psycho-social change appeared to have occurred with the introduction of dramatic activities for the participants, the workshop provided avenues for discussions on issues such as depression and drug abuse to hold. Indeed, as the medical Director of the hospital, Onuorah C. states "Basically, the inmates here have nothing much to do. There are not many activities that can engage them and on that front alone, this project could be very effective. Most of them are not different from you or I really. Many of them have similar stories of upbringing and the likes till something went wrong along the line. I sincerely think that these discussions should be held with members of the general public to educate those concerned better".

The applied theatre project thus endeavoured to fulfill the mandate of engendering inclusion and qualitative participation from the participants in further attempt to increase social interactions which was hitherto, not a predominant feature within the hospital. Indeed, the exclusivity as well as stereotypical connotations about inmates of the facility may have contributed to negative public perceptions and bias and these may have in turn had negative effects on the inmates themselves. The need thus, to utilize drama in educating the public on the various issues that could make any individual seek psychiatric medical evaluation and attention becomes imperative. The story of "Blessing", a 17 year old young mother who also participated in the project gives voice to this narrative. "Blessing" violently rejects her baby at the point of birth and is immediately taken to the Hospital. Indeed, while a number of reasons could be attributed to the sudden change in behavior among which, the medical director terms to be a "very acute case of post traumatic stress disorder", general perceptions and beliefs would rather point to factors such as "witchcraft", "diabolism" or "ancestral manipulations" as more believable reasons. Theatre could thus be effective in bringing these issues forward in a bid to provide community education among others. Yotis et al affirms that "Theatre methods have been used as instruments to promote inclusion of mental health patients in local communities and performance-making has proved to reduce prejudice and discrimination, promote health and build social networks. such methods can contribute to enhance community contacts, to promote community education and reach positive social change for adults living with psychiatric disabilities and their families".

The outcome from the Rehabilitation center in *Oredo*, however could be best described as progressive on a number of factors. While some of the participants who were physically challenged and made use of mobility aids such as wheelchairs, expressed continued interest and willingness for the course of the project, the other participants who were mainly comprised of mentally challenged children, were observed to not have increased significantly in positive psychosocial activities. The adoption of the story telling technique appeared to have engaged them to the extent of collaborative performance but not as much in the comprehension of messages needed for qualitative behavioural change.

The engagement of the rehabilitative potentials of Drama within formal systems of learning was brought to the fore in the *Ivbiore* and *Amaenyi* projects. Both projects evaluated the response of challenged school children in Nigeria to certain phenomena with relations to holistic psychosocial and cognitive development. The availability thus of the school "space" provided as an avenue practical and constructive knowledge could be created and/or learnt. The formal environment, the school provides also enables new trends of thoughts and actions to be learnt and assimilated. Mary Gauvain agrees when he observes that "Skill at solving complex problems in teams of people with varying backgrounds and expertise is needed to address many of the pressing social, environmental, health, resource and economic problems in the world today. There are several indicators of this new reality, social collaborative skills are increasingly valued and group work is seen as instrumental for tackling real world "grand challenge" problems and collaborative learning in the classroom is being used effectively for student learning across the curriculum".

The motive was not primarily to teach the pupils things they never knew but to work with them in putting concepts in perspective using the medium of Drama. Mbachaga states that "the core issue here is not feeding people with information in a top down model of intervention. The drama approach to education begins with what people know and works with them as subjects rather than objects to be handed information" (86). Similarly, the projects attempted to address challenges experienced by the participants while maintaining the ensemble nature that the dramatic arts possess. Theatre is a group art and entails the coming together of various individuals either as directors, actors, dancers, singers, props men, costume designers, drummers and so on in the creation of a performance or artistic production aimed at raising given issues about the human condition. However, it should be noted that though theatrical productions involve the participation and contribution of many people even with relations to applied theatre workshops, it also possesses the unique quality of allowing participants portray particular and peculiar perceptions borne out of individual or even collective experiences. All four projects engaged the participants from the standpoints of established communal as well as individual practices while employing activities and improvisational techniques in ensuring increased and sustained engagement and participation. The story creation and rehearsal processes thus, allowed participants to tell and reenact their own stories and as such allowing for needed conversations and action with other members of the community to be fostered.

Evaluations from the Projects

The applied theatre projects evaluated various given circumstances as well as individual experiences of participants within these localities. Some questions were administered prior to actual dramatic engagements to ascertain particular responses to communal behaviour as well as personal perceptions. The questions were designed to elicit responses needed to evaluated issues of self representation and worth, relationship with people, reception of new knowledge through the instrumentality of oral literature within the dramatic process and willingness to share their story and use same within a "play" context. These questions were also revisited as part of the post production evaluation.

In the school for the Blind project, 10 participants were fully engaged in the study; indeed all provided story material for the performance while some took part as actors, members of the orchestra and dancers. During the preliminary interactive sessions, a larger number of the participants expressed varied responses in the affirmative to questions bothering on whether discriminatory behavior from other people effected their sense of self worth. An example of the questions and solicited responses are:

Question: How do people's opinions of you make you feel?

Table 1

<table>
<tr><td colspan="2">Sometimes I feel it when someone doesn't want to be my friend so I stay on my own.</td><td colspan="2">I don't feel anything towards them. They are not God.</td><td colspan="2">I have heard people say things that are not true about me and some people believe them.</td></tr>
<tr><td colspan="3">I don't worry about other people opinion.</td><td colspan="3">I feel bad when people think that because I'm blind, I cannot do something meaningful.</td></tr>
<tr><td colspan="2">My teacher said it is because God knew I would be trouble, so he made me blind.</td><td colspan="2">Nothing. I still do what I want to do. I don't let it affect me.</td><td colspan="2">I really don't mind what is said about me.</td></tr>
<tr><td colspan="3">People quickly judge you sometimes without talking to you.</td><td colspan="3">Some people have said bad things, but people that know me, know I'm not like that so I'm ok.</td></tr>
</table>

The above responses indicate a general feeling of low self worth in the children interacted with. Some of the participants were indeed quite candid on issues of how other people's opinion about them affected them especially with regard to creating new relationships and adapting to new situations. The Applied Drama project allowed participants to express their views on the subject of bullying and discrimination in the various production meetings as well as in between rehearsals. When the same question was posed to the participants of the end of the production, the following answers were elicited.

Table 2

I have learnt that I am special and I can achieve what I desire despite people's opinion	People's opinion cannot define me.	I am happy with who I am. There are some talents I have to show the world.
I want to help people have a better understanding of people living with visual impairment.	I think I am in better control of my emotions.	
God has a purpose for me and I am going to fulfill them.	I wish people would stop hating people like me.	I will help them understand me more.
People will make you sad if you allow them. I choose to be happy.	I won't allow people to make me sad anymore because of my disability.	

The Amaenyi project engaged participants on similar issues as it concerns the menace of bullying and discrimination. Some of their sentiments were expressed before and after the production and noted below:

Question: How would you want people who have bullied and discriminated against you to treated?

Table 3

S/No	Before Dramatic Engagements	After Dramatic Engagements
P1	I wish that they become deaf and dumb so that they knew how it feels.	I forgive them. I will grow to be better so that they will know they were wrong.
P2	They should be arrested and put in jail.	
P3	I don't like remembering those things.	I pray they understand that I did not decide to be born this way.

P4	I don't even want to have contact with such people.	I forgive them, but I will not give them another opportunity.
P5	I leave them in the hands of God. Only they know why they do those kinds of things.	They should be taught that we are also human beings.
P6	Let their children suffer the same thing, then they would understand.	They should ask for forgiveness and know that what they are doing is wrong.
P7	They should be beaten up.	If they will listen, they should be taught better how to treat children with this disability.
P9	Let them be disgraced.	They should not be allowed to stay near children.
910	My aunty said that I'm possessed. She called me all sort of names. I prayed for it to happen to her child.	If it happened to her child, she won't be like that.
P11	If I could, I will make them like me for 1 week, then they will understand.	We should all be alive, they will see what I will become in future.

Observations revealed that prior to actual dramatic engagements, participants expressed general feelings of resentment and thoughts of retribution towards individuals that were found culpable of bullying children with hearing and speech difficulty. About six participants prescribed that such individuals be subjected to the same disabilities as appropriate punishment. These positions appeared to change as the project progressed. The infusion of dramatic enactments was aimed at developing and improving self worth to ensure that possible scenarios for discriminatory actions to occur are minimized.

Furthermore, a total of one hundred and twenty questionnaires were also distributed to adult-respondents within the Awka metropolis. As stated earlier, these questions sought to measure general perceptions on social attitudes towards the plight of children living with speech and hearing challenges as well as other forms of disabilities as they affect children and adolescents. Some of the responses retrieved are evaluated below:

Table 6: Do you agree that children with hearing and speech disabilities are more likely to be bullied and discriminated against?

S/N	RESPONSE	NUMBER OF RESPONDENTS	PERCENTAGE OF RESPONDENTS
1	YES	98	81.6%
2	NO	4	3.3%
3	MAY BE	18	15%
	TOTAL	120	100%

Table 7: Do you agree that spiritual forces could be responsible for hearing and speech loss in children?

S/N	RESPONSE	NUMBER OF RESPONDENTS	PERCENTAGE OF RESPONDENTS
1	YES	55	45.83%
2	NO	38	31.6%
3	MAY BE	27	22.5%
	TOTAL	120	100%

Table 8: Which of these do you think is more responsible for discriminatory actions meted out towards challenged children?

S/N	RESPONSE	FREQUENCY	PERCENTAGE OF RESPONDENTS
1	COMMUNAL/ RELIGIOUS PRACTICES	15	12.5%
2	INDIVIDUAL BEHAVIOUR	44	36.6%
3	BOTH	61	50.83%
	TOTAL	120	100%

CONCLUSION

The study set out to evaluate the impact of Theatre in addressing issues of psycho-social rehabilitation especially among at–risk children and adolescents. The thrust of the projects carried out attempted the utilization of Applied Theatre beyond the sphere of mere dramatic enactments, but in evaluating present issues experienced by challenged members of society with particular emphasis children and young adults. Indeed in the words Jenkeri Okwori, "Theatre can do more than entertainment. It can go beyond fiction to intervene in reality because it is based on it" (119). The study revealed that the selected projects in Ivbiore, Amaenyi, Oredo and Nawfia succeeded in forging inclusive modules for the teaching and learning of challenged children. The researcher's experiment fascinated the teachers and doctors who collaborated with the researcher and his team all through the experimental process.

It was also discovered that RehabDramatics has the potentials of rehabilitating psychologically traumatized challenged children. The experiment also broadened the scope of theatre-driven education. The several dimensions of applied theatre and therapeutic theatre is an over expanding area and have proved effective in this developing and rehabilitating at-risk children.

For children and young adults with special needs such as those studied within this research work. Applied dramatic activities also appear uniquely capable of engendering improved psychosocial change and development. Indeed, across the Applied Theatre projects carried out, there were attempts to particularize aspects of dramatic activities to individual participant challenges. The *Ivbiore* and *Amaenyi* projects engaged dramatic activities in addressing issues of bullying, negative stereotyping, low self esteem and so on. Participants were able to express themselves in the various activities which were geared towards achieving improved levels of self identification and representation. The *Oredo* project engaged story telling techniques embellished with dramatic performances to drive home needed messages on issues of peer bullying, the *Nawfia* project evaluated societal phenomena, such as depression, impact of drug abuse and Neglect, the infusion of dramatic art forms and other performative engagements encouraged increased psychosocial activities among participants. Indeed with sustained engagements, the dramatic art should continue to contribute as a therapeutic measure particularly in mental health intervention and studies. As Kristin Orjasaeter et al submits. "There is hope in practice and policy considerations that participation in arts project might have therapeutic benefits for people with mental illness and potential to facilitate key elements in mental health recovery. (2). Post production/follow up visits projected an increase in dramatic engagements in two out of the four communities visited namely the School for the visually impaired, *Ivbiore* and God's care special school, *Amaenyi* with the creation of performance groups in both places, to foster the continued engagements of theatrical activities and performances in dealing with disabilities.

Recommendations

The study recommends that more effort should be made to involve relevant stake holders such as parents, care givers, policy makers and indeed the general public on the need to engage inclusive and qualitative avenues of enhancing the quality of life of challenged children and adolescents. Indeed, there exists an apparent need to provide specialized and child-centered teaching techniques and care for children who suffer from different individual disabilities but who are often classified and diagnosed in group. Better attention should thus be paid to the different strands within these disabilities as this would further promote qualitative approaches in dealing with them. Average members of the community for example may not be able to easily distinguish between presentations of Attention Deficit Hyperactive disorder ADHD and General Anxiety Disorder GAD, in children or differences between Postpartum Depression and Schizophrenia in young adults and this may lead to incidents of wrong stereotyping which could eventually result to the formation of negative communal practices. Concepts such as RehabDramatics could be employed as interventionist measures in bringing to the fore the need to give particular attention and care to evolving challenges in today's child.

The study also recommends that Applied theatre concepts and techniques such as RehabDramatics should be engaged within the curriculum development of formal and non-formal educational establishments. These establishments such as primary, secondary and specialized centres of learning provide as important avenues of engaging developing children and as such, concepts like RehabDramatics could be instrumental in engaging challenged children on issues ranging from self representation to qualitative response to tasks and societal attitudes or practices. Similarly the study of Applied Theatre in Nigeria should be broadened in tertiary institutions to encourage more scholarly input in the area of Drama Therapy as a viable specialization area. This is to engender the utilization of the dramatic arts within multidisciplinary discourses and studies and thus encourage increased research interests particularly in the application of Theatre to health care delivery and practice.

Conclusion

It is hoped that the concept of RehabDramatics should contribute to the knowledge and practice of Applied Theatre research endeavours. Theatre as we have seen, possesses unique qualities in breaking boundaries of status, literacy, religion and so on. Applied dramatic concepts such as RehabDramatics thus, advocate for the integration of various art forms and performances with the aim of raising needed consciousness and activating discussions and actions towards productive change.

The need to continuously engage the community on social values, norms as well as established cultural practices using the dramatic medium provides as a viable alternative for theatre researchers and change agents. Indeed, until some of these practices are reenacted in a way that community members are brought in full glare of short or long term repercussions, many of the phenomena responsible for the seeming under-appreciation and underdevelopment of challenged individuals in society may continue unabated. It is therefore very likely that qualitative change in communal behaviour and attitudes could induce improved personal psycho-social responses that could foster better outlooks to life or as Levy Robb and Jindal Snape submit "Inclusive arts can support personalization in practice when it is conceived of from a social justice perspective (254). This inclusiveness as well as unique quality in engendering needed action, defines Applied Theatre techniques as a very effective medium.

RESEARCH PICTURES

Plate 12

Old & Newly erected sign post showing change of name from *School of the Blind* to *Special School for the Visually Impaired*

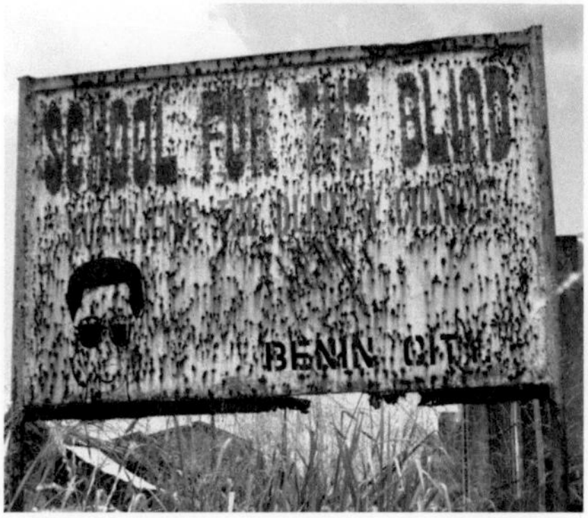

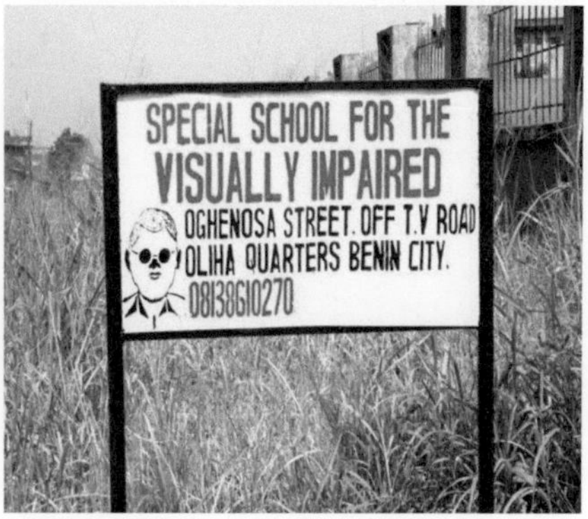

Post Production/follow up visit the HM of the Special School for the Visually Impaired and the representative from the Ministry of Education Edo State

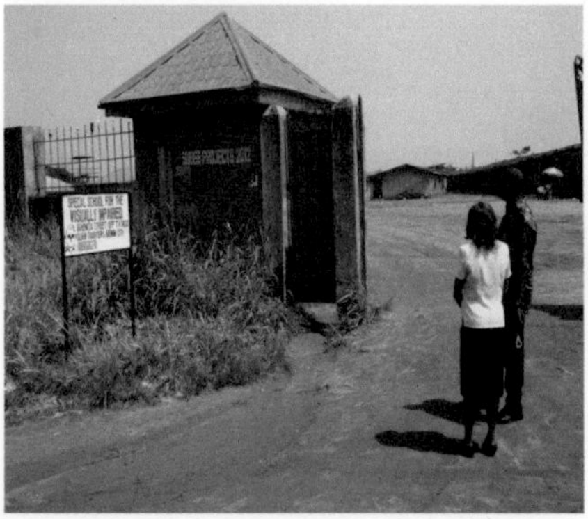

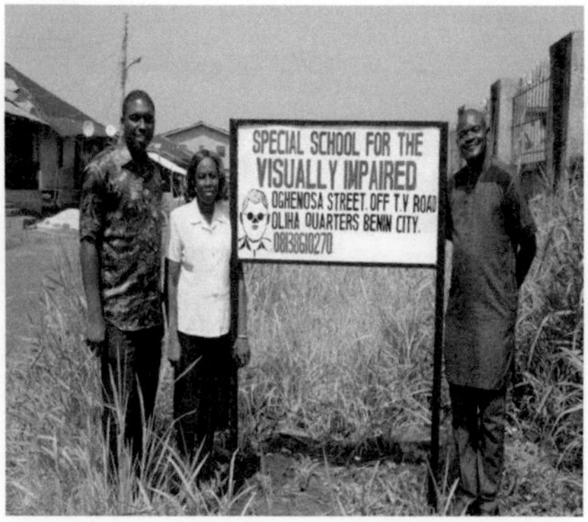

Plate 13

Infusing Performances to Validate Self Worth and self Representation with the Pupil "Miracle"

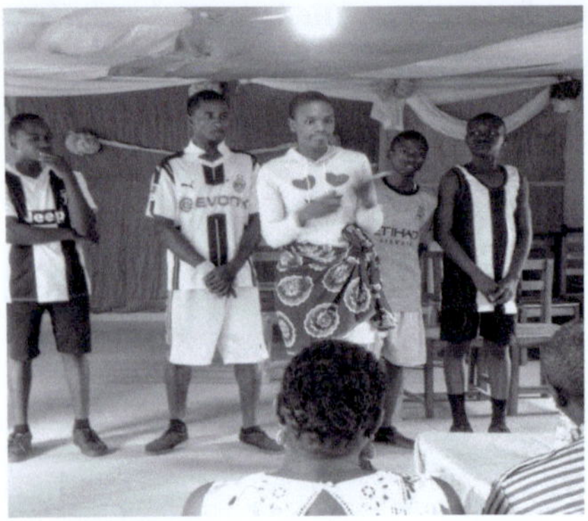

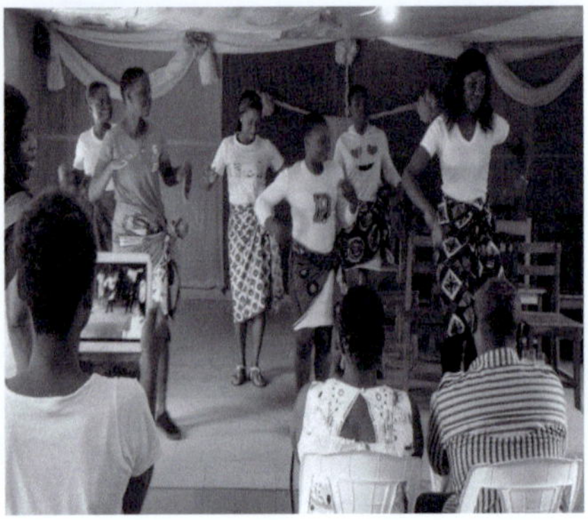

Using Drama in Addressing Issues of peer Bullying within and outside School Environment

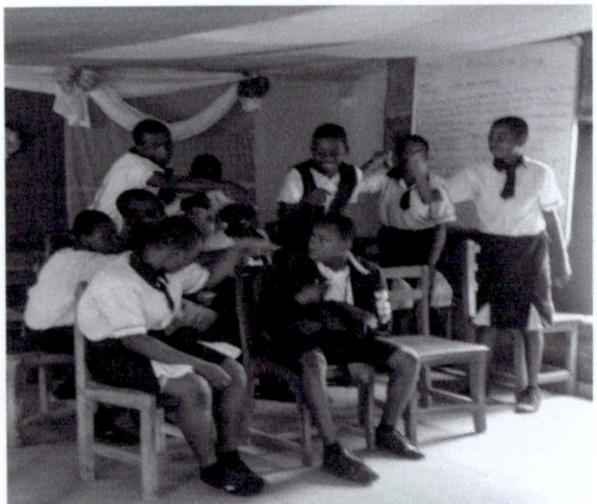

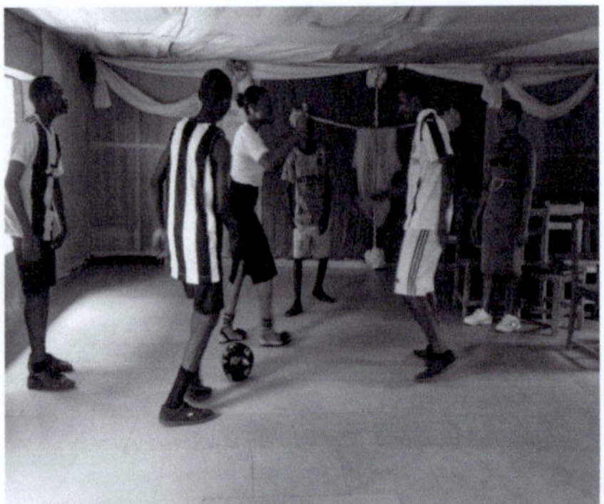

Plate 14

The Head Teacher and some Students of God Care Special School Amaenyi recounting what has been learnt from the Project

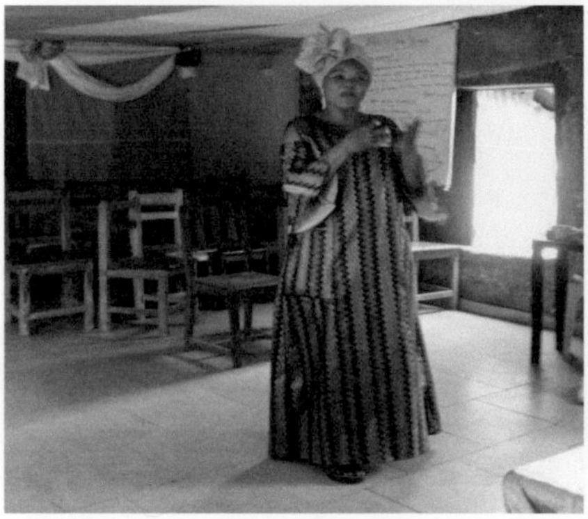

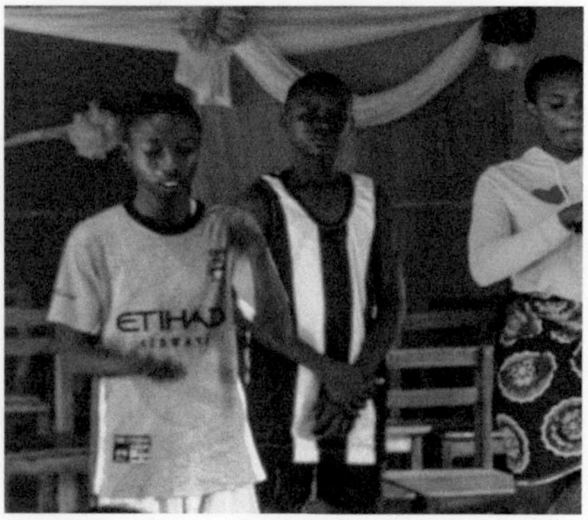

The researcher with the head teacher, Pupils and Research volunteers after series of rehearsals at God's Care Special School Amaenyi

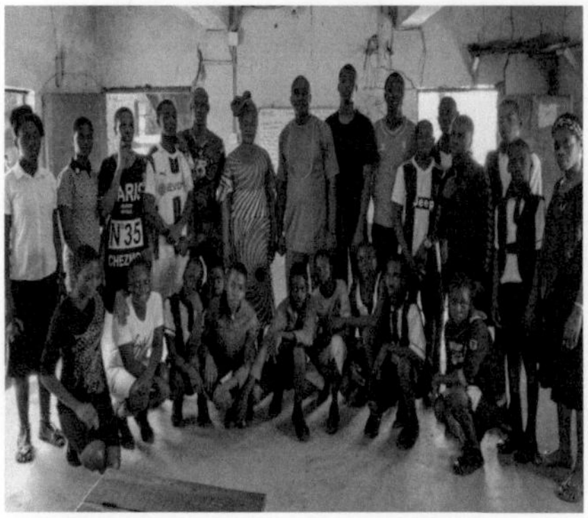

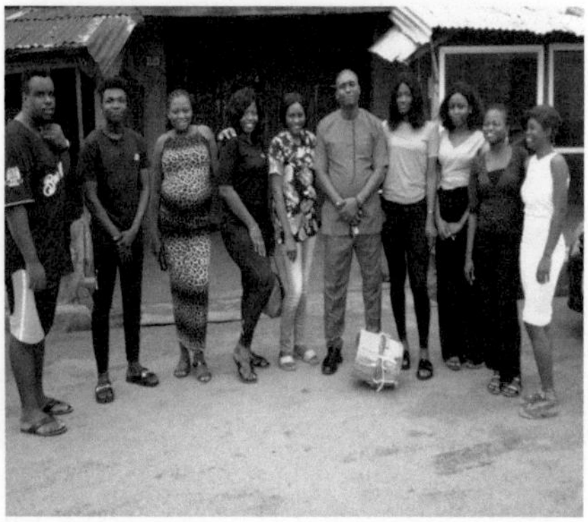

Plate 15

Dramatic enactments from the productions "Free" on how participants deal with depressive thought and situations

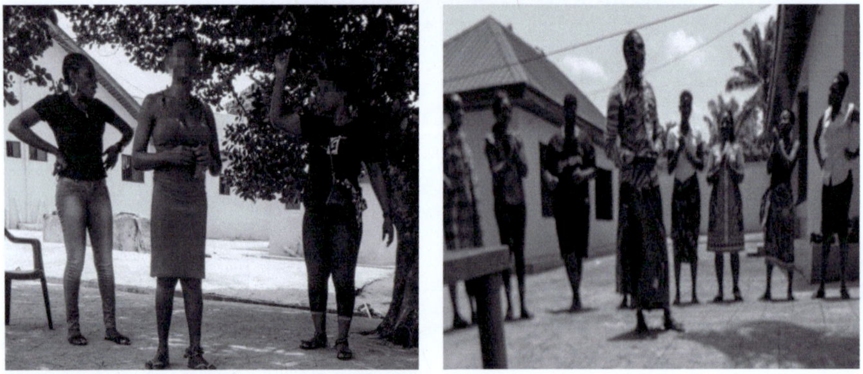

The menace of depression is represented in character of a bully who intimidates people into subjection. Depression is seen here challenging Blue Sky to a contest

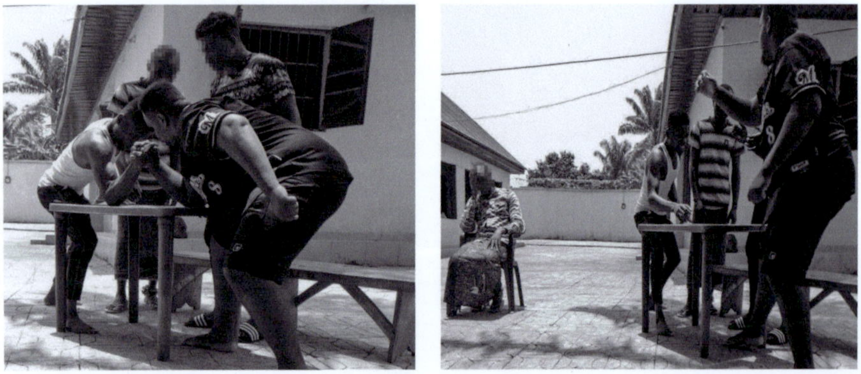

Plate 16

Blue Sky is encouraged and motivated by Members of his Community to defeat the bully (depression) after some attempts, he eventually succeeds

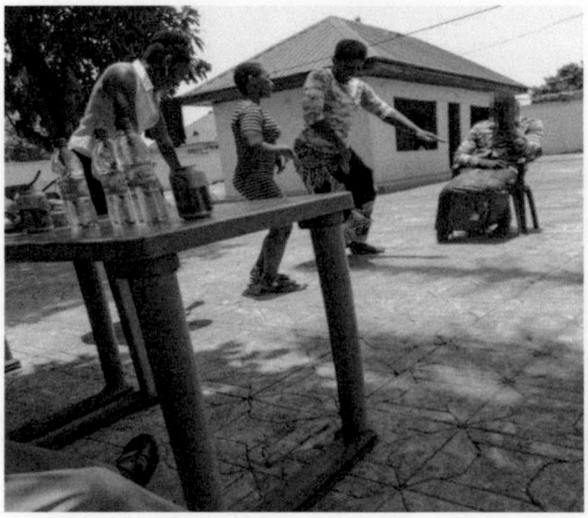

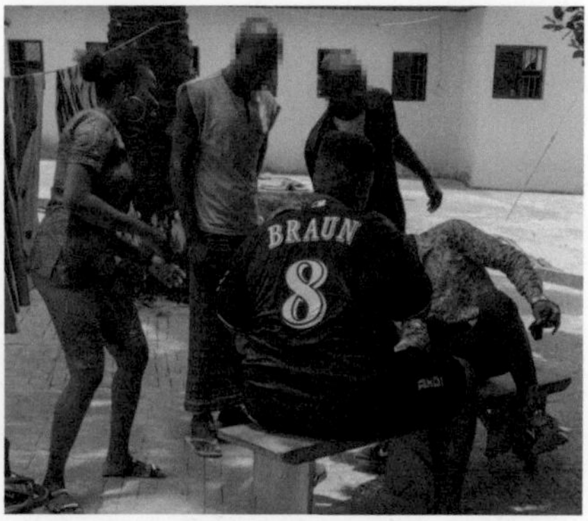

Post production interaction between "Blue Sky" and some of the research assistants on how the project has helped him

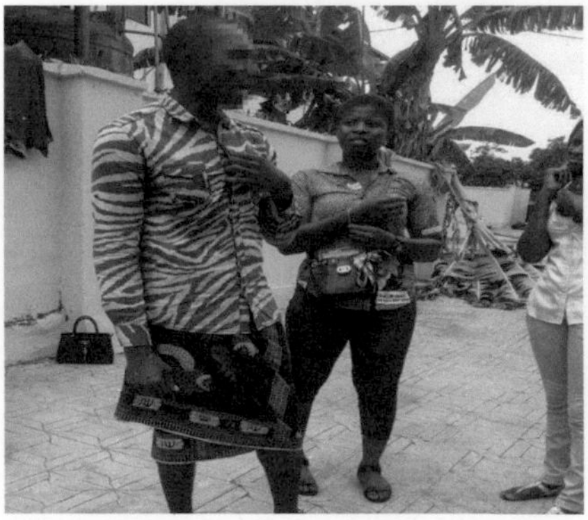

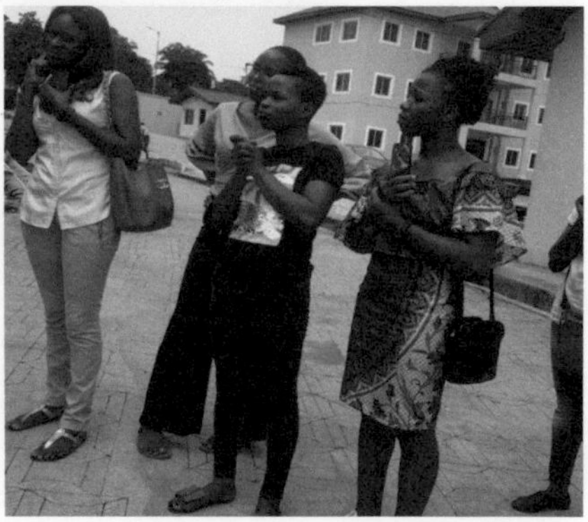

Plate 17

The researcher with his assistants/volunteers at the Nawfia Psychiatric Hospital, Anambra State

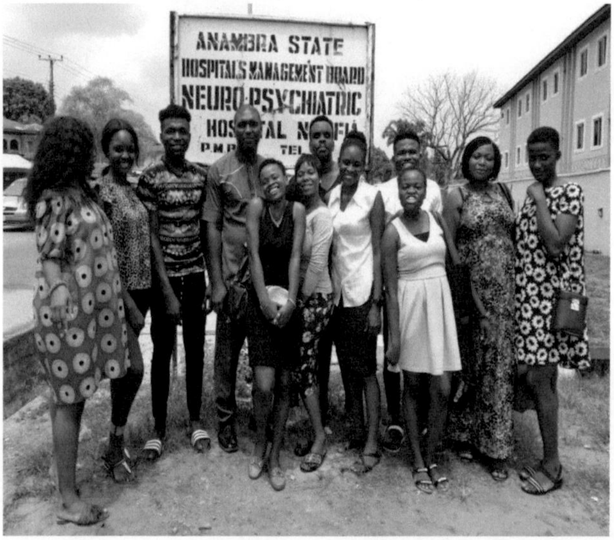

WORKS CITED

Agazue, Chima. Review of the book, "Spirit Children: Illness, Poverty and Infanticide in Northern Ghana". By Aaron R. Denham. *Criminal Law and Criminal Justice book Reviews*. 2017.

Allan, Robert and Eatough, Virginia. "The use of Interpretative Phenomenological Analysis in Couple and Family Therapy Research. *The Family Journal* Vol. 24 No 4 SAGE. London, 2016, 406 – 414.

Aradau, Claudia and Munster, Van Rens. "The Securitization of Catastrophic Events: Trauma, Enactment and Preparedness Exercises". Sage Publications, London, 2012:228-239.

Arinze-Umobi, Somto. "Adapting Folklore into Virtual Drama for the Nigerian Child's Education." *Journal of Theatre and Cultural Studies*. Vol. 8, No.1. AMA. Theatre Arts Department, Awka: Brystev and Publishers, 2013: 83-91.

Arpin, Jacques. "Masters of their Conditions II: Intercultural Theatre, Narration and Stage Work with Patients and Healers". *Transcultural Psychiatry*, Vol. 45, No 3. Geneva: SAGE Publications, 2008:355-378.

Bat'Or, Michal. Ishai, Rafi and Levi, Narkis,. "Validating PPAT'S Symbolic Meanings of Emotional and Cognitive Functioning among Children". *The Arts in Psychotherapy*, Vol. 41. Israel: Elsevier ltd. 2014:309-319.

Belliveau, G. "Engaging in Drama: using Arts-based Research to Explore a Social Justice Project in Teacher Education" International Journal of Education & the Arts, Vol7, No 5. 2006: 127-148.

Bolton, Gavin. Towards a Theory of Drama in Education London. Longman Group limited,1979.

Bosco, N., Petrini, F., Giaccherini, S., Meringolo, P. "Theatre as Instrument to Promote Inclusion of Mental Health Patients. An innovative experience in a local community in C. Pracena. *Psychological Application & Development*. Lisboa: Science press. 2014: 55-66.

Brown-Shaw, Muriel. Westwood, Marv and De Vries, Brian. "Integrating *Personal Reflection and Group-based Enactments". Journal of Aging Studies*, Vol. 13, No. 1. Vancouver: JAI Press. 1999:109-119.

Butler, Elmien Bakker, M. Terri and Viljoen Gerhard. "Poetic and Therapeutic Encounters in an Adolescent Drama Group". *South African Journal of Psychology*, Vol. 43. No. 1, SAGE; Pretoria, 2013:94-104.

Cassidy, Susan, Turnbull, Sue and Gumley, Andrew. "Exploring Core Processes Facilitating Therapeutic Change in Dramatherapy: A Grounded Theory Analysis of Published Case Studies." *The Arts in Psychotherapy*, Vol. 41. UK: Elsevier ltd. 2014:353-365.

Chae, Soo Eun and Kim, Soo Jin. "Group Psychodrama for Korean College Students." *Journal of College Student Psychotherapy*, Vol. 31, No. 1, New York; Routledge, 2017:59-70.

Chin-lee, Tsung. "Trilogy of Body Imagery: Dance/Movement Therapy for a Psychmatric Patient with Depression". *The Arts in Psychotherapy* Vol. 41. Taiwan: Elsevier ltd. 2014:400-408.

Chukwunwem, Bramwell. Director Salvation Army Rehabilitation Center, Oredo Benin City. Oral Interview. 19th Oct. 2018.

Clarke, Robert. "Divorce in Nigeria: Things fall Apart." The Economist July 7th 2016. Accessed 13th Sept. 2018.

Cohen, Czamanski J. Sarid, O. Huss, E. Ifergane, A and Niego, L. "CB-ART-The use of a Hybrid Cognitive Behavioural and Art Based Protocol for Treating Pain and Symptoms Accompanying coping with chronic illness." *The Arts in Psychotherapy*, Vol. 41. Israel: Elsevier ltd. 2014:320-328.

Cohen, Orna and Heinecke, Andreas. "Dialogue Exhibitions: Putting Transformative Learning Theory into Practice." Curator: *The Museum Journal*. Vol. 61, No.2. France: Wiley periodicals inc. 2018:269-283.

Combs, Charles. "Theatre and Drama in Education" http.ericdigest.org// creative.html assessed April 26th 2017.

Courtney, R. Play, Drama and thought. The Intellectual Background to Drama in Education. New York; Drama Book Specialists Publishers, 1989.

Crawford, Paul, et al, eds. "Health Humanities: The Future of Medical Humanities." *Mental Health Review Journal*, Vol. 15 No. 3.UK: Pier Professional ltd 2010.

Curnow, Joe. "Fight the Power: Situated Learning and Conscientisation in a gendered Community of Practice." *Gender and Education*. Vol. 25, No. 7, Toronto: Routledge. 2013:834-850.

Curtis, Anne. "Communicating with Bereaved Children: A Drama Therapy Approach." Principles & Practice: Illness, Crises and Loss Vol.7, No 2. New York: 1999, 183 – 190.

Dima, Gabriela and Bucuta, Mihaela D. "The Method of Interpretative Phenomenological Analysis in Pschodrama Research". *HAUPTBEITRAGE, Psychodrama Soziometr*, Vol. 15. Romania: Springer ltd. 2016:69-81.

Dogan, Turkan. "The Effects of Psychodrama on Young Adults' Attachment Styles." *The Arts in Psychotherapy*, Vol. 37, Ankara; Elsevier, 2010:112-119.

Emunah, R. Acting for Real: Drama Therapy Process, Technique and Performance. New York: Brunner/Mazel,1994.

Eren, Nurhan, Ogunc, Nazan Emil and Keser, Vehbi. "Psychosocial, Symptomatic and Diagnostic Changes with Long-term Psychodynamic Art Psychotherapy for Personality Disorders". *The Art in Psychotherapy* Vol. 41. Istanbul: Elsevier ltd. 2014: 375-385.

Erskine, Richard, "Relational Group Process: Development in Transactional Analysis Model of Group Psychotherapy." *Transactional Analysis Journal* Vol. 43 No 4. Sage Publications Vancouver 2013: 262 – 275.

Ezenwa-Ohaeto. "Subject, Context and the Contours of Nigeria Fiction." *African Studies series*, Ibadan; Pia Theelmann and Eckhard Breitinger, 1995.

Ezenweke, Elizabeth. O. "Good Governance and the Dynamic of Eschatology: African Traditional Religious Experience Humanities and Good Governance. Faculty of Arts, Awka: Rex Charles and Patrick Ltd, 2012: 267-273.

Fayose, P.O. A Guide to Children's Literature for African Liberians and Parents. Ibadan: AENL Educational Publishers, 1995,

Fisher, Robert. "Thinking about Thinking: Developing Metacognition in children." *Early Child Development and Care*, Vol. 141 No. 1. Malaysia: Routledge. 1998:1-15.

Gauvain, Mary. "Collaborative Problem Solving Social and Developmental Considerations" *Sage Journals*. New York, accessed No 29, 2018.

Gbenga , Rotimi. "folklore as a Source of Material for Educational Theatre in Secondary Schools for Cultural Reconstruction." Proceeding of the 27th Annual convention and Int'l Conference of the Society of Nigeria Theatre Artists, Lagos. 2014:34-45.

Gbinigie, Florence. Former Commissioner for Women Affairs and Social Development. Edo State. Oral Interview. 7th Nov. 2018.

Gile, Krista .J. and Handcock, Mark .S. "Respondent Driven Sampling: An Assessment of Current Methodology." *Sociological Methodology*, Vol. 40. No. 1. Oxford: Nihm. 2010:285-327.

Gstrein, Dorathea. “Effectiveness of Psychodrama Group Therapy on Pupils with Mathematics Anxiety”. *Zeitschrift Fur Psychodrama and Soziometrie*, Vol. 15. Italy; Springerlink.com. 2016:197-215.

Haneda, Mari. “Classrooms as Communities of Practice. A Re-evaluation.” *TESOL Quarterly*, Vol. 40, No. 4. Ohio: www.jstor.org. Accessed 02-09-2018:807-817.

Hans-Gerd, Ridder. “The Theory Contribution of Case Study Research Designs.” Vol. 10 issue 2, University of Harmonar, Germany. Springer Books, 2017: 281 – 305.

Heckwolf, Jessica I. Bergland, Christy and Mouratidis, Maria. “Co-ordinating Principles of Art Therapy and DBT”. *The Arts in Psychotherapy*, Vol. 41. USA: Elsevier ltd. 2014:329-335.

Howie, Pter and Bagnall, Richard. “A Beautiful Metaphor: Transformative Learning Theory.”*International Journal of Lifelong Education*, Vol. 32, No. 6, Australia: Routledge. 2013:816-836.

Idede, Blessing H/M School of the Blind. Ivbiore. Benin City. Oral Interview. 8th Nov. 2018.

Idogho, A.J “Drama in Education for Sustainable Children Development.” *AMA: Journal of Theatre and Culture Studies*, vol8. 2013: 121-

Illeris, Knud. The Three Dimensions of Learning. Malabar, Fla: Krieger Pub Co, 2004.

Illich, Ivan. Deschooling Society. New York: Harper & Row 1970.

Immigration and Refugee Board of Canada “Nigeria: Divorce Law and Practices among Christians, Including Grounds, Procedures Length of Process, Property Disposition, Child custody and Consequence for the Woman and her family. Published 2 Nov. 2012. http://www.refworld.org/docid/. Accessed, 13th Sept. 2018.

Jackson, Tony *Learning through Theatre*. London: Routledge, 1993.

Jakobson, Roman and Bogatynev, Petr. “Folklore as a Special form of Creation.”http://scholarworks.iu.edu. Accessed 9/4/2019.

Janik, D.S Unlock the Genius Within. Lanham, Md: Rowman and Littlefield education, 2005.

Johnson, Andrew P. “How to use Creative Dramatics in the Classroom Academic Journal Article Childhood Education, 1998. http://www.questia.com. Accessed 24/9/2019.

Jones, P. Drama as therapy, New York Routledge, 2010.

Kalisa, Chantal "Theatre and the Rwandan Genocide; Art from Trauma: Genocide and healing beyond Rwanda University of Nebraska Press USA Accessed 6/8/2019 from http://bookgoogle.com.ng

Kilinc, Sultan. Farrand, Kathleen, Chapman, Kathryn and Kelly Michael. "Expanding Opportunities to Learn to Support Inclusive Education through Drama Enhanced Literacy Practices." *British Journal of Special Education*, Vol. 44, No. 4. UK:NASEN ltd. 2017:431-447.

Kim, Jihyun. Kim, Gabsook and Seo, Sohee. "Validation of the FSA as Screening Tool for children with ADHD." *The Arts in Psychotherapy*, Vol. 41. Korea: Elsevier ltd. 2014:413-423.

Kitchenham, Andrew. "The Evolution of John Mezirow's Transformative Learning Theory." *Journal of Transformative Education* Vol. 6, No 2. Canada: SAGE Publications. 2008:104-123.

Korthagen, Fred. A.J. "Situated Learning and the Pedagogy of Teacher Education: Towards an Integrative View of Teacher Behaviour and Teacher Learning." *Teaching and Teacher Education Journal*, Vol. 26. Amsterdam: Elsevier ltd. 2009: 98-106.

Lamont, Scott Brunero, Scott. Development of an Interactive Multimedia Mental Health Education Program for Generalist Nurses." *Collegian: Sciverse Science Direct*. Sidney: Elsevier ltd. 2013:239-247.

Lave, J and E, Wenger. Situated Learning Peripheral Participation New York: Cambridge Press, 1991.

Leonard David, *Learning theories, A to Z*. Westport. Conn: Oryx press, 2002.

Levy, S. Robb, A. J. and Jindal-snape, D. "Disability Personalisation and Community Arts: Exploring the Spatial Dynamics of Children with Disabilities Participating in Inclusive Music Classes." *Disability and Society*, Vol 32 No 2. Dundee UK. Routledge 2017: 254 - 268.

Mantecon, A. Juan, M. and calafat, A. "Respondent Driven Sampling: A New Sampling Method to Study Visible and Hidden Population. *Adicciones*, Vol. 20, USA: pubmed.gov.2003.

Mbachaga, D.J. "Drama and Safer Sex Education Among Secondary School Teenagers in Benue State. *Nigerian Theatre Journal*, Vol. 10, No 1. JOS: SONTA. 2010:83-95.

McCaslin, Nellie. Creative Drama in the Classroom and Beyond. 6th ed. New York: Longman Publishers, 1996.

McLeod, S. A. "Piaget: Cognitive Stages of Development" accessed 24 Jun, 2018. http:www.simplypsychologyoro/piaget.html

Michel, A., & Oyduk, O. "Willpower in Cognitive Affective Processing system." Handbook of *Self-regulation; Research Theory and application*. New York: The Guilford, 2014: 99-129.

Morris, J. Frances. "Should art be Integrated into Cognitive Behavioural Therapy for Anxiety Disorders?". *The Arts in Psychotherapy*, Vol. 41. USA: Elsevier ltd. 2014:343-352.

Muleka, Joseph. "Theory in the Study of African Oral literature; The oral Artist's Agenda". *Journal of Arts & Humanities*. Vol. 3, No. 7. University of Nairobi, Kenya: MIR, 2014: 85-91.

Nagner, Bettyjane. *Building Moral Community through Educational Drama*. Stanford, Connecticut: Ablex Publishing Corporation, 1999.

Normann, Nicoline; Lonfeldt, Nicole Nadine and Reiholdt-Dunne, Maria Louise. "Negative thoughts and Metacognitions in Anxious children following CBT". *Cogn ther Res*, Vol. 40, New York: Springer Media ltd. 2015:188-197.

Nwosu, C.C "Patterns of Socio-economic Change and Child Development in Africa: A paper presented at the 2nd Global conference. Mansfield College Oxford, United KingdomJuly, 2012.

Obadiegwu, C. "Educational Theatre and Qualitative Inquiry: The Unizik Experience." *AMA Journal of Theatre and Cultural Studies*, Vol. 4, 2009: 27-46.

Obadiegwu, C. Play for Transformation: Reflections on Classroom Drama for Learners Empowerment. Awka: Eunique Press, 2019..

Obadiegwu, C. "Performative Empowering Pedagogy and Transformative Students' Development." *Journal of Theatre and Cultural Studies*. Vol. 1, No. 1. 2012.

Odimegwu, Ike. "Globalisation and the African Identity: Towards a Universalist Reconceptualisation" ed. M. Asiegbu and J. Agbakogba, Ibadan: Philosophy and Praxis, 2006.

Okwori, Jenkeri. "Empowering the disempowered; Using popular Theatre for rural transformation in Nigeria." Case Studies in Practice of Theatre for Development. Zaria; Tamanza publishing company, 2005

Olusakin, Mopelola. A. *et'al* "Towards Helping children with Attention Deficit Hypererative Disorder (ADHD) to Enjoy Preschooling". Study Home comm.. University of LagosOnline Journal, 2008.

Omoko, Peter .E. "Themes of Environmental despoliation and Social Injustice in Urhobo Popular Songs." *The Creative Artist*. Vol. 7 No. 2: ed. Tracie Utoh-Ezeajugh, Awka: Valid Publishing Company, 2012: 1-11.

Onogu, Williams .S. "Folk Media and Rural Development in Nigeria: Implication for Development Theatre." *Nigerian Theatre Journal*, Vol. 10, No.1 Jos: SONTA 2010: 65-72.

Onuorah, C.C. Medical Director/Consultant in-charge, Neuro Psychiatric Hospital Nawfia, Anambra State. Oral Interview. 15th Oct. 2018.

Onwuegbuna, Ikenna. "Philosophical Embodiment in Igbo Music: An Analysis of Mike Ejeagha's "Popular" "Folk Songs Styles" Creative Commons/Sage Open.uk 2015, 1 – 7.

Orjaesaeter, Kristin Berre. Davidson, larry. Hedlund, Marianne. Bjerkeset, Ottar. Ness, Ottar. "I now have a life." Lived Experiences of Participation in Music and Theatre in a Mental Health Hospital: Page One Vol 13 (12). University of Twente, Netherlands: December 2018.

Orkibi, Hod and Azoulay, Bracha. "Adolescents' Dramatic Engagement Prediction. In-session Productive Behaviours." A Psychodrama Change Process Study: The Arts in Psychotherapy, Vol. 55, Elsevier. Israel, 2017:46-53.

Osterlind, Eva. "Drama in Higher Education for Sustainability: Work Based Learning through Fiction?" *Higher Education, Skills and Workshop Learning*. Vol. 8, issue 3, Sweden Emerald insight publication. 2018:337-352.

Otueroro, Onome. Director of Publicity, Conference of non Governmental Organizations (CONGOS) Upper Sakponba, Ikpoba Okha, Benin City, Edo State. Oral Interview. 7th Nov. 2018.

Ozbek, A., and Leutz, G. Psychodrama; Enactment Interaction in group psychotherapy. Ankara: Has-Soy Printing House. 1987.

Pammenter, David. "Devising for TIE" Learning through Theatre ed. By Tony Jackson. Theatre, New York. Routledge. 1993:53-70.

Piaget, J. *Construction of Reality in the Child*. London: Routledge and Cegan Paul, 1957.

Pickup, Ian. "Child-centered Teaching Methods Enhance Early Childhood Physical Education. Accessed 10th September 2018 from"http://www.humankinetics.com/excerpts/child-centredteaching.

Pien, D. and Rothbert M.K *Incongruity and Resolution in Children Humor: A Re-examination of Child Development* Vol.9, Oxford: Blackwell Publishing, 1960.966-971.

Ratsoy, Ginny R. "Class Participation in an Aboriginal Theatre Project: An Exemplar of Undergraduate Student Engagement". *The Canadian Journal for the Scholarship of Teaching and Learning*. Vol. 2. Issue 1. Scholarship@ western.2011.

Rousseau, Cecile; Beauregard, Caroline and Daignault, Katherine. "A Cluster Randomized-controlled Trial of a Classroom-based Drama Workshop Program to Improve Mental Health Outcomes among Immigrant and Refugee Youth in Special Classes". *PLOS ONE Journal*, Vol. 9, issue 8. Canada: cross mark. 2014.

Schissel, Dana "What is child development? Definition, theories & stages" www.study.com/us.coursesNavigator.accessed 3/10/2018.

Silius-Ahonen, Ellinor and Gustavson, Maria. "To Learn and not to Learn-that is the question". *Procedia-Social and Behavioral Sciences*, Vol. 29. Helsinki: Elsevier ltd. 2011:809-818.

Sullivan, John. Petronella, Sharon. Brooks, Edward and Murillo, Maria. "Theatre of the Oppressed and Environmental Justice Communities: A transformational Therapy for the Body Politic". *Journal of Health Psychology*, Vol. 13. No 2. Texas: SAGE Publications. 2008:166-179.

Tassoni, P and Hucker, K. Planning in Early Childhood. Oxford. Heinemann educational Publishers, 2005.

Taylor, Edward .W. Transformative Learning Theory. Wiley periodicals Inc. Pennsylvania; 2008.

The British English Dictionary, Oxford University Press. 1989

The Online Etymology Dictionary. http://www.dictionary.com/definition. thesautus.com accessed, 24/9/2019

Transformative Learning centre. The transformative centre Toronto: Canada. Retrieved September 23, 2018, www.http://tic.oise.utoronto. Ca/index. htm.

Tsu, Gary and Bannerman, Brittany. Transforming Trauma into Healings and Being: a Non-Dual therapy Approach International Journal for Mental Health Addiction, Vol. 15, New York: Springer science media. 2016:63-79.

Utoh – Ezeajugh, Tracie. "Theatre and Contemporary Realities; The Dynamics of social change in Nigerian Plays". Theatre Experience, Journal for Contemporary Theatre Practice. Vol. 1 No. 1 Awka: Penmark Publishers 2002: 123 – 134.

Vygotsky, L. Mind in society. Cambridge, Ma: Harvard University Press. 1978.

Wenger, Etienne Communities of Practice: Learning, meaning and identity. Cambridge, UK: Cambridge University Press, 1998.

Wenger, Ettenne. "Communities of Practice and Social learning systems". Organization Articles, Vol. 7. No. 2. London: SAGE Publications. 2000:225-246.

Wertsch, J.V. from Social interaction to higher psychological processes: A clarification and application of Vygotsky's theory, New York, sharpe Publ. 2008.

White, David "Social Phenomena: Definition and Examples" http//study.com. chapter 9 lesson 31, accessed 8 March, 2019.

Yaniv, Dan. "Revisiting Moravian Psychodramatic encounter in light of contemporary neuroscience: Relationship between empathy and creativity". The Arts in Psychotherapy, Vol. 38, Isreal Elsevier, 2011:52-58.

Yotis, Layo. Theocharopoulos, C. Fragiadaki, C. and Begioglou, D. "Using Playback Theatre to address the stigma of mental Disorder". The Arts in Psychotherapy, Vol. 55, Athens; Elsevier, 2017: 80-84.

Zanchetta, Margareth Santos. Bailey, Annette and Kolisnyk, Olesya. "Mentors' and Mentees' intellectual-partnership through the lens of the transformative learning Theory". Nurse Education in practice, Vol. 25. Toronto: Elsevier ltd. 2017:111-120.

Zimmerman, B.J Theories of self regulated learning and academic achievement: An overview and analysis Hillside, New Jersey: Erlbaum, 2001.

APPENDIX 1

DEPARTMENT OF THEATRE AND FILM STUDIES. NNAMDI AZIKIWE UNIVERSITY, AWKA.
PMB 5025, AWKA, ANAMBRA STATE, NIGERIA

Okoye Chukwudi Michael
(Reg. No. 2015107011P)
Department of Theatre and film studies,
Nnamdi Azikiwe University, Awka.
15th Oct. 2018

Dear Respondent,

Below are questions needed to aid the research work on the engagement of RehabDramatics and the Development of Challenged Children and Young adults. The answers provided will be utilized for educative purposes only and the researcher assures of the non-disclosure and indemnity of your personal information and details.

Your co-operation is most appreciated.

A) Demographic Column

1) Gender Male ☐ Female ☐
2) Age Bracket 10 – 15 ☐ 16 – 25 ☐ 26 – 35 ☐ 35 – above ☐
3) Occupation, specify e.g student, civil servant, business man etc
   ....
4) Are you a parent?
5) Are you related to someone living with disability?
   i) Yes ☐ No ☐
   ii) Specify relationship ....
   iii) Specify the type of disability ....

APPENDIX 2

DEPARTMENT OF THEATRE AND FILM STUDIES. NNAMDI AZIKIWE UNIVERSITY, AWKA.
PMB 5025, AWKA, ANAMBRA STATE, NIGERIA

External Memorandum

To: H/M School for the Blind, Ivbiore, Benin City, Edo State. **Date:** 15th Oct. 2018	**From:** Okoye Chukwudi Michael (Reg. No. 2015107011P Department of Theatre and film studies, Nnamdi Azikiwe University, Awka. Approved for 3 months

APPLICATION TO USE YOUR SCHOOL FOR THE RESEARCH ON THE UTILIZATION OF APPLIED THEATRE ACTIVITIES THROUGH REHAB DRAMATICS AS AN INTERVENTION MECHANISM FOR CHILD DEVELOPMENT

I wish to apply for the above subject matter in your establishment.

This research work is basically aimed at integrating the applied drama approach to the discourse of child learning and development. The study discusses in detail the potential of dramatic activities not just as an entertainment or educative tool but as being capable of rehabilitating at risk children by engendering improvement in psychosocial skills and development healthier responses to environmental issues situate in Nigeria.

The study will be relying on a number of theories and concepts in the actualization of the research work. They are the situated learning theory,

the theory of Transformative learning, The Psychodramatic approach to development, the theory of metacognition and self regulation and the African Oral literary tradition.

The researcher in course of this research work intends to carry out interactive and enactment with 20 children between the ages of 10 – 15 and engage the concepts of Theatrical spontaneity through games, play and so on to ascertain levels of dramatic self representation in dealing with the present realities of problem solving as experienced by traumatized or at risk children and adolescents in Nigeria.

The study is purely for research purposes only and as such the identities and privacy of the participants will be well protected.

For your kind consideration.

Yours faithfully,

Chukwudi Michael Okoye.

SCHOOL FOR THE BLIND

DATE 08-11-18

BENIN CITY

APPENDIX 3

DEPARTMENT OF THEATRE AND FILM STUDIES. NNAMDI AZIKIWE UNIVERSITY, AWKA.
PMB 5025, AWKA, ANAMBRA STATE, NIGERIA

External Memorandum

To: Chief Medical Director Psychiatric Hospital Nawfia, Njikoka LGA, Anambra State. **Date:** 15th Oct. 2018	**From:** Okoye Chukwudi Michael (Reg. No. 2015107011P Department of Theatre and film studies, Nnamdi Azikiwe University, Awka. approved for 4 months

APPLICATION TO USE YOUR HOSPITAL FOR THE RESEARCH ON THE UTILIZATION OF APPLIED THEATRE ACTIVITIES THROUGH REHAB DRAMATICS AS AN INTERVENTION MECHANISM FOR CHILD DEVELOPMENT

I wish to apply for the above subject matter in your establishment.

This research work is basically aimed at integrating the applied drama approach to the discourse of child learning and development. The study discusses in detail the potential of dramatic activities not just as an entertainment or educative tool but as being capable of rehabilitating at risk children by engendering improvement in psychosocial skills and development healthier responses to environmental issues situate in Nigeria.

The study will be relying on a number of theories and concepts in the actualization of the research work. They are the situated learning theory,

the theory of Transformative learning, The Psychodramatic approach to development, the theory of metacognition and self regulation and the African Oral literary tradition.

The researcher in course of this research work intends to carry out interactive and enactment with 20 children and young adults between the ages of 15 – 20 and engage the concepts of Theatrical spontaneity through games, play and so on to ascertain levels of dramatic self representation in dealing with the present realities of problem solving as experienced by traumatized or at risk children and adolescents in Nigeria.

The study is purely for research purposes only and as such the identities and privacy of the participants will be well protected.

For your kind consideration.

Yours faithfully,

Chukwudi Michael Okoye.

Received
Dr. C. C. Onuorah
Consultant-in-charge

STATE HOSPITALS
MANAGEMENT
NEUROPSYCHIATRIC
HOSPITAL NAWFIA

APPENDIX 4

DEPARTMENT OF THEATRE AND FILM STUDIES. NNAMDI AZIKIWE UNIVERSITY, AWKA. PMB 5025, AWKA, ANAMBRA STATE, NIGERIA

External Memorandum

To: Director Salvation Army Rehabilitation, Center No 20, First East Circular Road, Oredo LGA Edo State. **Date:** 15th Oct. 2018	**From:** Okoye Chukwudi Michael (Reg. No. 2015107011P Department of Theatre and film studies, Nnamdi Azikiwe University, Awka. Approved for 3 months

APPLICATION TO USE YOUR CENTER FOR THE RESEARCH ON THE UTILIZATION OF APPLIED THEATRE ACTIVITIES THROUGH REHAB DRAMATICS AS AN INTERVENTION MECHANISM FOR CHILD DEVELOPMENT

I wish to apply for the above subject matter in your establishment.

This research work is basically aimed at integrating the applied drama approach to the discourse of child learning and development. The study discusses in detail the potential of dramatic activities not just as an entertainment or educative tool but as being capable of rehabilitating at risk children by engendering improvement in psychosocial skills and development healthier responses to environmental issues situate in Nigeria.

The study will be relying on a number of theories and concepts in the actualization of the research work. They are the situated learning theory,

the theory of Transformative learning, The Psychodramatic approach to development, the theory of metacognition and self regulation and the African Oral literary tradition.

The researcher in course of this research work intends to carry out interactive and enactment with 20 children between the ages of 10 – 15 and engage the concepts of Theatrical spontaneity through games, play and so on to ascertain levels of dramatic self representation in dealing with the present realities of problem solving as experienced by traumatized or at risk children and adolescents in Nigeria.

The study is purely for research purposes only and as such the identities and privacy of the participants will be well protected.

For your kind consideration.

Yours faithfully,

Received by Major Bramwell. Chukwuanwem. 19/10/2018

SALVATION ARMY
REHABILITATION CENTRE

Chukwudi Michael Okoye.

APPENDIX 5

DEPARTMENT OF THEATRE AND FILM STUDIES. NNAMDI AZIKIWE UNIVERSITY, AWKA.
PMB 5025, AWKA, ANAMBRA STATE, NIGERIA.

External Memorandum

To: Director God's Care Special School Umuayom, Amaenyi Awka South LGA, Anambra State. **Date:** 15th Oct. 2018	**From:** Okoye Chukwudi Michael (Reg. No. 2015107011P Department of Theatre and film studies, Nnamdi Azikiwe University, Awka. Aproved for three months

APPLICATION TO USE YOUR SCHOOL FOR THE RESEARCH ON THE UTILIZATION OF APPLIED THEATRE ACTIVITIES THROUGH REHAB DRAMATICS AS AN INTERVENTION MECHANISM FOR CHILD DEVELOPMENT

I wish to apply for the above subject matter in your establishment.

This research work is basically aimed at integrating the Applied drama approach to the discourse of child learning and development. The study discusses in detail the potential of dramatic activities not just as an entertainment or educative tool but as being capable of rehabilitating at-risk children by engendering improvement in psychosocial skills and develop healthier responses to environmental issues situate in Nigeria.

The study will be relying on a number of theories in the actualization of the research work. They are the Situated learning theory, the theory of Transformative learning, The Psychodramatic theory, the theory of Metacognition and self regulation and the African Oral literary tradition.

The researcher in course of this research work intends to carry out interactive and enactment sessions with 20 children between the ages of 10 – 15 and engage the concepts of Theatrical spontaneity through games, play and so on to ascertain levels of dramatic self representation in dealing with the present realities of problem solving as experiences by traumatized or at-risk children in Nigeria. The researcher will also engage the Interpretatative Phenomenological Approach as a Qualitative research instrument in ascertaining progress levels of the study.

The study is for research purposes only and as such the identities and privacy of the participants will be well protected.

For your kind consideration.

Yours faithfully,

Chukwudi Michael Okoye.
08034499914

Mrs Ndife I.B
Proprietress
17/6/2019